Sustaining Persons, Grieving Losses

Sustaining Persons, Grieving Losses

*A Fresh Pastoral Approach
for the Challenges of the Dementia Journey*

DIANNE CROWTHER

FOREWORD BY
NEIL PEMBROKE

CASCADE *Books* • Eugene, Oregon

SUSTAINING PERSONS, GRIEVING LOSSES
A Fresh Pastoral Approach for the Challenges of the Dementia Journey

Copyright © 2017 Dianne Crowther. All rights reserved. Except for brief quotations in critical publications or reviews, no part of this book may be reproduced in any manner without prior written permission from the publisher. Write: Permissions, Wipf and Stock Publishers, 199 W. 8th Ave., Suite 3, Eugene, OR 97401.

Cascade Books
An Imprint of Wipf and Stock Publishers
199 W. 8th Ave., Suite 3
Eugene, OR 97401

www.wipfandstock.com

PAPERBACK ISBN: 978-1-4982-3795-6
HARDCOVER ISBN: 978-1-4982-3797-0
EBOOK ISBN: 978-1-4982-3796-3

Cataloguing-in-Publication data:

Names: Crowther, Dianne Elizabeth. |

Title: Sustaining persons, grieving losses : a fresh pastoral approach for the challenges of the dementia journey / Dianne Crowther, with a foreword by Neil Pembroke.

Description: Eugene, OR: Cascade Books, 2016 | Includes bibliographical references and index.

Identifiers: ISBN 978-1-4982-3795-6 (paperback) | ISBN 978-1-4982-3797-0 (hardcover) | ISBN 978-1-4982-3796-3 (ebook)

Subjects: LCSH: Pastoral care | Dementia | Dementia—Religious aspects—Christianity | Dementia—Patients—Religious life| Care for the sick—Religious aspects—Christianity

Classification: BV4435.5 C87 2017 (print) | BV4435.5 (ebook)

Manufactured in the U.S.A.   JANUARY 17, 2017

This book is dedicated to my beloved parents, and to all who travel this journey with courage.

Table of Contents

Foreword by Neil Pembroke ix
Preface xiii
Acknowledgements xv

Introduction xvii
Chapter 1. Grounding Care: Sustaining Persons in Context 1
Chapter 2. Grounding Pastoral Care: Spirituality and Meaning 17
Chapter 3. Caregiving: A Lived Experience 30
Chapter 4. Caregivers' Journeys: Themes and Meanings 67
Chapter 5. Grieving Losses: "The Long Goodbye" 100
Chapter 6. Local Pastoral Practice, Perspectives, and Meanings 117
Chapter 7. Theological Foundations for Care 154
Chapter 8. A Pastoral Approach 177
Chapter 9. Moving Forward 190
Epilogue 197

Appendix A: Guidelines for Caregiver Interviews 201
Appendix B: Local Practice Study 205
B. 1: Email to Church Leaders
B. 2: Focus Group Discussion Questions

Bibliography 209
Index 217

Foreword

THERE ARE A VARIETY of drivers behind the writing of a work of pastoral theology. Sometimes it's as pragmatic and utilitarian as meeting a demand from a Head of School to get some published work out or lose your job! Pastoral theologians, like other academics, need to publish to survive. There is no doubt about what motivated Di Crowther to write her wonderful book, *Sustaining Persons, Grieving Losses*. Di cares deeply about improving the care that is offered to persons on the dementia journey. When one reads relevant reports from churches in the North from the eighties and early nineties, a similar picture emerges. Church leaders of the time acknowledged that the exclusion of people with dementia was a pressing problem. In the intervening period, some improvements have been made, but there is a long way to go. The fact that Di had so much trouble getting local church leaders to engage with her research project says something. As she puts it, it was very evident that care of people on the dementia journey is generally viewed as "a low priority." That's profoundly sad. It also points to the fact that the work that Di Crowther has done is vitally important and desperately needed.

Di's approach is multi-disciplinary. She begins by providing a careful and thorough survey of the work done in the human and social sciences on care of people with dementia. She expresses appreciation for Kitwood's very helpful subject-to-subject relational care model. I also resonate strongly with his approach. In my own pastoral theology, the dialogical philosophy of Marcel and Buber has played a central role. The I-Thou relation is at the very heart of faithful and effective caregiving. John Swinton, in his theological reflection on relational care, identifies the sacramentality of the experience of deep connection in the stillness of presence and love. It is this perspective that takes us to the core of Di's approach.

Di extends the theological reflection by turning to the doctrine of the Trinity. There was a time when pastoral theologians would run a mile from this doctrine. What help, they wanted to know, could the arcane, abstract, convoluted thinking that theologies of the Trinity serve up possibly offer us? Not too many pastoral theologians think like that anymore. The doctrine of the Trinity has undergone a massive revival in the theological world over the past thirty years. Di picks up on this and sets up a very important and illuminating conversation between the intersubjective approach of Kitwood and others, on the one hand, and trinitarian theology, on the other. She notes that the doctrine that we humans are made *imago Dei* can be further explicated: we are made *imago Trinitatis*. That means that ontologically we are persons-in-communion.

Di's work is thoroughly theological. It is also grounded through empirical research. In order to sharpen her sense of the emotional and spiritual challenges faced by caregivers, she listened to the stories a select group of them were ready to tell her. Further, she investigated current pastoral practice through work with focus groups. Di listened intently for the "gaps and silences" to inform her thinking.

One of the gaps is that caregiver grief is commonly neither sufficiently understood nor appropriately acknowledged. She very helpfully identifies "anticipatory grief" and "ambiguous loss" as the major challenges. Di here hits upon a very important missing piece of the jigsaw puzzle. Of all of the elements in her model, none is more crucial than this one.

Every practical theologian knows that the work is not done upon completing a description of current practice and doing critical correlational theology. The ultimate aim in one's research is renovation of practice. With this in mind, Di concludes her research by providing a comprehensive, practical, and deeply insightful model of care for those on the dementia journey. She is completely right in her judgment that there are five essential elements required for a comprehensive new approach to pastoral care of persons with dementia and their caregivers. Those elements are education, advocacy, inclusive worship, an inter-church support program, and liaison and cooperation with the broader community. The way in which she discusses these areas is full of insight on the one hand, and eminently practical on the other.

Di Crowther has done us all a wonderful service in offering us her thorough research and profoundly helpful insights. I join with her in her fervent hope that those who read this book will capture the vision and offer the quality pastoral care that persons on the dementia journey too often have missed out on. The fact that many people suffering from dementia

Foreword

have experienced exclusion is tragic. Through her research, Di has made a very significant contribution to the vitally important and urgent task of turning things around.

Neil Pembroke,
University of Queensland, 14 March 2016.

Preface

MY INTRODUCTION TO DEMENTIA was as an adult daughter experiencing the long-term journey of my mother's forgetting, my father's caring until his death, and the continuing journey beyond that. In the midst of other challenges and other layers of ambiguous loss and unacknowledged grief, I was largely unaware of my emotions. I was fully occupied with coping—until one day, on the way home from a visit with my mother in the aged care center, the emotions came tumbling out as deep grief. Eighteen months later when she died, no grief flowed, and I felt robbed.

A little later, in my role as an aged care and community chaplain, I was deeply blessed and enriched through connecting with many persons with dementia and family caregivers. I share the following vignettes which capture precious splashes and bitter drops of the essence of their journeys.

Eva, for fifty years the gentle loving wife of William, talked with me following one of her daily visits to William in the dementia unit of the aged care center. She expressed her deep and unfulfilled yearning for her husband to put his arms around her again. She confessed to me, rather apologetically, that she had expressed that longing to her son, a "wonderful Christian," only to be brought back to reality rather sharply by her son's response: "Oh Mum, don't be silly! You lost your husband years ago. Get over it." Eva said to me, in a tone both pleading and slightly defiant, "But I haven't, have I? Because he's still here!"

In my chaplaincy role I regularly visited Charles, a very elderly retired Christian minister living in the community. We shared conversation, prayer, and the Lord's Supper together many times, as the irregular visits from his church became more and more widely spaced. As his forgetfulness increased, so his will to live diminished. I would find him huddled in his chair, shrunken and hopeless in his losses and aches, wishing life would end. After hearing his struggles, I would remember with him his life of faith and service, and he would gradually connect with who he had been and who he still was. We would share the Lord's Supper, and he would often conclude with a prayer ringing with confidence. When I left, he would be standing with his back straight, his head high, and a wide smile on his weather-beaten face, sustained in the presence of the God he had served faithfully, as a loved child of the Father.

Faith was a retired Christian missionary, with no family. She had been a resident for years in an aged care center. She was no longer mobile, and no longer had verbal communication. She spent her days semi-reclined in her chair, and life was quiet for her. I used to visit her, and would sit quietly holding her hand as we held each other's gaze, and we would be together in the peace of the moment. I would read a brief Scripture, and we would share the Lord's Supper. And her smile is one of the sweetest memories of my chaplaincy years.

At a community event I had a brief chat with a minister whom I had previously seen at times conducting a Eucharist Service for his denomination, in the "Sunnyside" Aged Care Centre where I was chaplain. Before bustling off to speak to someone else, he said, "Oh, we don't visit there anymore. There are none of our people there now—oh, except Caroline of course, so there's no point." Caroline had been a long-term member of his congregation, and had participated in the Eucharist service led by him at "Sunnyside" for some years after moving there. She had been rather proud of her church and her life, but was now slipping graciously into forgetfulness, simplicity, and grace. On my regular visits, she would reminisce over her early life or we would be still together, quietly enjoying the birds and the sweep of the lawn outside her window. At the conclusion of a visit more than a year after my conversation with her minister, following our prayer in which she participated, I gave her the customary kiss on her forehead. She reflected, "When you kiss me, I think of it as Jesus kissing me. He's here, you know."

The unstated questions hang in the air: Why bother with pastoral care for those facing the challenges of dementia? Why use precious and stretched church resources—those people are catered for by community care and health services and Alzheimer's support groups, are they not? And they have their family. There are plenty of people in the congregation facing major issues, so why bother with those people who will not remember? What is the point? And anyway, it's the young people we need to focus on, is it not?—they're our future!

Acknowledgments

My deep thanks go to my husband Noel, whose moral support encouraged me to undertake this task, whose practical support kept life flowing so that I could complete it, and whose spiritual support has been with me all the way.

I gratefully acknowledge Neil Pembroke's contribution to this work, through his generous encouragement and his wisdom, and through introducing me to the joys of practical theology. I acknowledge the support both he and Ray Reddicliffe offered me throughout my PhD, the forerunner to this work. I thank my good friend Ruth Williams, who read this manuscript with great care and insight, and gave her feedback with love.

I am grateful for the literature now available on supportive dementia care, and deeply indebted to John Swinton for his contribution of a theology of dementia, which has challenged, enlightened, and inspired me.

I am deeply grateful to the participants in the caregiver study, who, in the midst of their taxing journey, gave me their precious time, and opened their lives and hearts to me. My gratitude goes also to the participants in the local practice study, who put aside their busy schedules to contribute invaluable insights into their churches' and their own pastoral responses to the dementia journey.

For the compassionate and deeply committed people with whom I have worked in aged and community care, who relate to and love their residents and clients as valued persons, I have heartfelt respect and appreciation. To the many who have shared their journey with me, some into forgetfulness, some through long grief, and many into a space of sacred intimacy where we knew that God was with us, I offer my thanks. It has been an amazing privilege to walk the path with you, and see God's love on your faces and in your stories; you have touched my heart deeply and enriched my life profoundly.

Acknowledgments

My deepest praise and gratitude go to God, who opened the door and led me onto and along this path. It has been my joy, in every nook and cranny and turning of the path, to discover that God, the God who is love, is there before me.

Introduction

DEMENTIA, INCLUDING ALZHEIMER'S DISEASE and other conditions associated with diminishing cognitive functioning, is recognized as a major health and social issue of the twenty-first century, impacting on the lives of increasing numbers of people in aging populations. A person's experience of dementia is recognized to be significantly affected by the social environment and the quality of care provided. Family caregivers, usually the primary contributors to this quality of care while persons with dementia live at home, face extremely stress-provoking challenges; and if a person enters a residential aged care center, the family caregiver generally continues to maintain ongoing relational connection while facing a new set of caregiving challenges.

The well-being of those facing the challenges of dementia first-hand and those who care for them is, then, a pressing issue; and the need for a multidisciplinary approach to dementia care is increasingly acknowledged within the social and health sciences. While health services and community service providers may offer physical and social care, and organizations such as Alzheimer's Association may provide practical information and some emotional support, the need for ongoing emotional and spiritual care is often overlooked in service provision. This underlines the importance of a relevant Christian pastoral response, first to members of Christian communities who face the dementia journey, and then to those in the broader community who travel the road without adequate support.

The discipline of practical theology undertakes reflective critical enquiry into the practice of the church in the world, in the light of God's purposes and in dialogue with cultural sources of knowledge. It has dual roles: practical, responding to the real needs of our world, and theological, seeking to "regain the transcendent appeal of God's word to humanity."[1] It is

---

1. Veling, *Practical Theology*, 18.

Introduction

contextual, paying careful attention to a particular phenomenon in order to deepen understanding of the situation and practice, and it is theologically reflective, with the aim of developing new theory that is worked out in practice and that reflects what we understand to be God's purposes. We attend, then, to the real experience of human beings, and ask searching questions about "gaps and silences" that should be addressed in life situations,[2] questions that we seek to answer with integrity and in practice, questions such as:

> Who has a complaint against us? With this question we raise the issue of who is cared for and who is not. Who is served? . . . Who finds a voice? Who remains silent? . . . And most importantly, whose burden is multiplied by the way we go about our business?[3]

For some time there have been expressions of concern from Christian ethicists, pastoral theologians, and pastoral caregivers about attitudes in churches towards persons with dementia and their care. Indeed, in the UK back in 1990, a Church of England report noted that "Christian theology and the practice of the church . . . seem tacitly to exclude the person with dementia."[4] Since that time, core theological, ethical, social, and pastoral issues around dementia have been addressed, and there is a small but growing body of literature on the subject of Christian pastoral care for persons with dementia and their caregivers. However, anecdotal evidence and written accounts of both caregivers and persons with dementia raise serious questions about the extent to which that tacit exclusion has been replaced by caring and relevant pastoral practice informed by the theological and cultural insights of the intervening decades.

Being both practical and theological from the outset, the task of developing an appropriate approach to pastoral care fits within the field of practical theology. We explore what Christian response is called for and on what theological grounds, to what extent available knowledge—both pastoral and cultural—is currently informing practice in this area of pastoral care, and how we might bridge the gap between our theological rhetoric of care and our pastoral practice towards persons facing the challenges, losses, and grief of dementia. Indeed, we ask how we might, as Christian community,

---

2. Pattison with Woodward, "Pastoral Theology," 42.
3. Thornton, *Broken yet Beloved*, 116.
4. *Ageing: Report*, 91.

Introduction

participate in this journey so that the burden may be lightened as persons are sustained in the compassionate love of God and in the body of Christ.

Pastoral care that seeks to be Christian must be grounded in the church, and in the Scriptures and rigorous Christian theology;w and at the same time it must take account of the situation it addresses and the needs of those it seeks to nurture. To inform our understanding of the current situation and thinking, we explore relevant literature from cultural and pastoral sources concerning the emotional and spiritual needs of those facing ongoing memory loss and those who care for them. In this process, we engage in dialogue between contemporary theory and practice from the social sciences and relevant theological themes, where each informs the other. This dialogue is approached unapologetically from the position that the Christian Scriptures and tradition are the norm and guide in faithful Christian discipleship and compassionate care. We also explore the actual experience of caregiving, and pastoral practice in one geographical location. In response to the insights gained in this descriptive phase, we reflect theologically on what constitutes an appropriate Christian pastoral response, with a view to building up communities of faith as they seek to care for their own members and to reach out with care to the vulnerable in the wider community. The process thus moves towards an enhanced practice responsive to the perceived needs, and reflecting a normative Christian perspective.

First, then, we explore the current knowledge and thinking around dementia care. It is important to consider the foundations and approaches to care as articulated within the fields of the human and social sciences. Recent developments in person-centered, supportive, relational care for persons with dementia are based on an understanding of personhood bestowed through human relationships. This concept invites dialogue with theological themes of relational, embodied personhood bestowed by God, where the spirit is seen to touch all aspects of life. Psycho-social understandings of identity and the importance of relationships for its sustenance inform and challenge Christian pastoral practice. Current broad understandings of spirituality and religion are considered, and connection, meaning-making, and transcendence are found to be common threads. We argue that spiritual care takes its place within "whole-person" care, and explore literature relating to the spiritual and religious needs and care of those facing the challenges of dementia.

Introduction

The description of the present situation is broadened by empirical research, firstly into the experience of caregiving. We hasten to acknowledge that the experiences of persons with dementia are no less important than those of caregivers, and that further empirical studies with persons with dementia are needed. However, in view of the importance of relationships and the social context for the well-being of persons with dementia, an understanding of caregivers' experiences and needs is vital in supporting both caregivers *and* those for whom they care. The experience of a small number of caregivers is explored through an interpretive phenomenological research study. We hear the stories of six caregivers who are at different points in the journey from diagnosis to the year following the loved one's death, and noteworthy themes that emerge through a year of their individual experiences are analyzed interpretively. An overall thematic analysis of the experience of these caregivers is offered, and the findings are considered in the broader context of theory and research. The study reveals something of the emotional and spiritual challenges of individual caregivers, and their expectations and experience of support; and although, of course, these experiences do not represent the full range of challenges, they do give "on-the-ground" insights into the journey.

Moving from the grief-imbued stories of these particular caregivers, grief theory in relation to dementia is reviewed and developed. While grief is increasingly acknowledged to be a major factor in the dementia journey, there are gaps in understanding and in services addressing this issue. From within the social sciences there are ongoing calls for further research into the complex grief of caregivers and persons with dementia, and for relevant grief interventions to be initiated and evaluated. We explore recent bereavement grief theories for their applicability, and consider literature relating specifically to the grief of caregivers and persons with dementia. Through this process it becomes evident that meaning-making offers common ground: as an approach for processing grief, and as a spiritual task. A spiritual framework is therefore argued to be appropriate for the development of grief interventions for the dementia journey. Within this framework, spiritual care offers opportunities for the enfranchisement and processing of grief, for making meaning in grief and in life, for nurturing the identity and personhood of both caregivers and persons with dementia, and for transcending the challenges.

Having discussed the needs and heard the pain of the journey, we broaden the description of the phenomenon through exploring some current Christian pastoral approaches, as a starting point in developing an appropriate pastoral response. We examine "on-the-ground" pastoral practice relating to dementia and grief, in order to understand what is being done and what "gaps and silences" there may be in practice. Qualitative research has been undertaken, by means of a focus group study, into pastoral practice in relation to those on the journey within Christian churches in a particular Australian locality. Representatives of all accessible churches in this locality were invited to contribute to the research through participation in a focus group. Here, they were invited to describe their churches' practices in response to the needs, discuss their challenges in this pastoral ministry, and suggest theological and other resources that were or might be helpful. Findings give an indication of what is being done pastorally in this locality. It must be noted that these two empirical studies are small-scale and exploratory, and seek to illuminate the broader context rather than to produce findings that claim to be universally applicable. The ensuing insights inform the development of an approach to pastoral care for the journey.

Finally, we engage in theological reflection on themes arising from the theoretical and empirical findings, and move toward enhancing pastoral practice. Themes include Christian community that reflects the interdependence of the "body" metaphor of 1 Corinthians 12; *agape* love, hospitality, and friendship; solidarity in suffering, lament, and hope; identity and meaning-making; and prayer and worship in the context of Christian community. The proposed approach to pastoral care addresses the need for healthy Christian communities where *all* are cared for, the equipping of faithful spiritual companions for individuals and families facing the challenges of dementia, and an initiative offering emotional, relational, and spiritual support for those on the journey in churches and the broader community. To these ends, we propose education, advocacy, and an interchurch support program.

This approach, then, responds to the needs identified in experience, theory, and literature; and it invites the expression of the faithful, relational love of God. Thus we seek to hear those who may often be unheard, to offer care that lightens rather than increases the load of those traveling the road, and, together in the community of the loved, to love and sustain persons grieving the losses of the often-long journey through dementia.

1

Grounding Care: Sustaining Persons in Context

Those whose personhood we have had the temerity to question may be the very persons to teach us to see our own personhood in a fresh light and to lead us to re-evaluate human possibility.
—John Killick, "Magic Mirrors"

As we seek to offer Christian pastoral care to persons with dementia and their family caregivers, we need to understand whom we are supporting, on what grounds, and by what means—in other words, *whom*, *why*, and *how*. Within the field of practical theology, it is almost universally recognized that a critical engagement with cultural sources leads to more informed and well-rounded theology and practice. Important themes in dementia studies include personhood, identity, and relational context; and if pastoral care is to be supportive of persons with dementia and those who care for them, we must take account of what we can learn from the human and social sciences in these areas. However, we begin with theology, rather than neurology or medicine or psychology, to provide the context and offer the larger story—indeed the counter-story—of dementia: that we as human beings are created by God, we reside in creation as embodied, en-spirited, and relational persons with a personhood that cannot be lost, and we live in the love from which we cannot be separated.[1]

This chapter, then, begins by addressing the theme of the person from moral, sociological, and theological angles. These perspectives raise the

1. Swinton, *Dementia*, 17–20.

question of the status of persons with dementia—whether they are "lesser," "lost," or "remembered" persons. We argue for the theological concept of an irrevocable personhood bestowed by God, and sustained in relationship with God and other persons. We explore and listen to cultural approaches to the provision of care for persons with dementia—person-centered, supportive, relational, communicative, empathic care. Such approaches seek to sustain persons and to build a positive counter-story in the face of malignant social positioning and stereotyping. We acknowledge the importance of the relational context for persons with dementia; and we identify challenges faced by caregivers in this journey. Thus we begin to lay the groundwork for an appropriate pastoral response to the challenges faced in the dementia journey.

The Person

The Moral Challenge

Among a range of disciplines including theology, ethics, sociology, and psychology, there are those who point out that the care of persons with dementia is inextricably tied to a society's values and concepts of personhood. The ethicist Stephen Post argues that the moral quality of a civilization depends in part on how people with dementia and other cognitive impairments are treated, and he asserts that in an individualistic, rationalistic, productivity-focused society, the primary task of dementia ethics is to affirm a common humanity as the basis of respect.[2] He notes that in our hyper-cognitive culture "the dictum 'I think, therefore I am' is not easily replaced with 'I will, feel, and relate while disconnected by forgetfulness from my former Self, but still, I am.'"[3] Others echo the concern that rationalistic, hyper-cognitive values are reflected in dehumanizing attitudes toward persons with cognitive impairment. Such attitudes include seeing a person with one impairment as wholly deficient, assuming that persons with dementia do not experience emotional suffering, and categorizing persons and reducing them to the generic, rather than recognizing them as

---

2. Post, "*Respectare*," 224.
3. Post, *Moral Challenge*, 3.

individuals.[4] As Stokes succinctly puts it, "dementia for most of the twentieth century was denied a human face."[5]

In recent decades, sociological and gerontological theory and research have challenged such depersonalizing attitudes, and have responded with new approaches to caring for persons with dementia. Kitwood, in seeking to overturn the prevailing "malignant social psychology," challenged attitudes toward persons with dementia that resulted in stigmatization, exclusion, invalidation, banishment, objectification, disparagement, and the less visible *sheer neglect* that deprived people of meaningful human contact.[6] Moving away from the earlier paradigm of the medical model of people with dementia as objects to be "warehoused," Kitwood was instrumental in establishing a new paradigm, wherein the person rather than the condition became the focus.[7] His understanding of personhood as "a standing or status that is bestowed upon one human being, by others, in the context of relationship and social being"[8] has become the basis for recent person-centered approaches to dementia care.

However, such a definition calls for careful analysis. As Dewing argues, implicit in this is a "secondary status of personhood" conferred on persons with dementia by others.[9] Swinton elaborates this further, noting the precarious nature of personhood with such a foundation.[10] He argues that if personhood has to do with only temporal relationships, "then what we are as persons will inevitably become unraveled as our relational networks break down."[11] If human beings have the power of bestowal of personhood through relationship, they equally have the power of withdrawal of this status through withholding relationship and care; and the personhood of each of us is at the mercy of the choices of others. The search for a more enduring foundation for "person-centered" care invites dialogue with theology.

---

4. Sapp, "Ethics and Dementia," 358–61.
5. Stokes, "Psychological Interventions," 159.
6. Kitwood, *Dementia Reconsidered*, 45–49.
7. Ibid., 7–9.
8. Ibid., 8.
9. Dewing, "Personhood: Revisiting," 6–9.
10. Swinton, *Dementia*, 149–52.
11. Ibid., 149.

A Theological Understanding

From a theological perspective, to understand dementia is to begin from a different starting point, from a concept of personhood in the context of creation. Trinitarian theologians see the *imago Dei* as the foundational concept for a biblical understanding of the nature and value of personhood, for "to be a person is to be made in the image of God."[12] Gunton sees the being of God as consisting in personal communion, where the persons of the Trinity share a common divine nature as discrete persons existing eternally only in a relationship of love, bestowing on one another particularity and freedom.[13] He argues that we are beings created in the image of God to be in relationship with God, with a horizontal dimension in relationships where "like God, but in dependence on his giving, we find our reality in what we give to and receive from others in human community."[14] Certainly, we need to question theological approaches that begin with social theory, move to project human ideals onto God, and then reflect that understanding of a relational Trinity back to be the basis of our understanding of human relationships.[15] Nonetheless, the reexamination by contemporary theologians of the biblical understanding of the Trinity highlights the relational essence of the *imago Dei*.

We begin, then, not by defining personhood in terms of capacities or human relationships, but in terms of a "way of being" as created, relational persons, from which capacities and relationships emerge through the embodiedness of human beings born into the human family.[16] As Swinton says:

> Personhood thus relates to the way that human beings are in the world and relate in and to one another and the world. It is not a set of capacities, and it is not simply a standing that is bestowed upon someone by others. It is an irrevocable status that comes from being a human being.[17]

Such a theological understanding of God's bestowal of personhood—a status wholly determined by God, who continuously reaches out in love to

---

12. Gunton, *Trinitarian Theology*, 116.
13. Ibid., 117–19 for the extended argument.
14. Ibid., 117.
15. Kilby, "Perichoresis and Projection," 441–43.
16. Swinton, *Dementia*, 155–59.
17. Ibid., 157.

human beings created in God's image—offers a secure foundation for a personhood nurtured through relationship with God and relationships with other human beings. It also offers a challenge as to how we see and relate to all other persons in the world, including those with cognitive impairment.

Sustaining Persons

Lost Persons?

There is ongoing discussion around the implications of personhood, identity, and the self in dementia. In lay discourse, there is often a focus on the "disappearance" of the "true" person, with terms such as "loss of the person," "loss of identity," and "loss of self" featuring prominently.[18] Recent dementia research concerning the grief of caregivers has focused on loss, and has in some instances included the concept of relating to the person who has been, rather than the person who is there now. This loss perspective is also expressed by people with dementia themselves. Snyder quotes a participant in her research: "it isn't the death. It's the loss of oneself while you're still alive."[19] Family caregivers, in writing of their experience, express similar perspectives: "grieving over the loss of my father's identity. . . . He is this different man—a lost person wandering through the wilderness."[20] Shenk speaks of the fear of Alzheimer's as "the fear of losing your identity while your healthy body walks on into oblivion."[21] As Killick suggests, there is a "weighty body of theory and attitude against the maintaining of selfhood in dementia."[22]

Remembered Persons

The question of what constitutes our identity is interesting and challenging. Swinton points out that our memory is subjective, saturated with emotions, complex, unreliable, and open to distortions; and if we are equating memory with identity, our own identity too, is open to question.[23] He ap-

---

18. See Killick, "Dementia, Identity," 60–61 for examples of such writings.
19. Snyder, *Speaking Our Minds*, 72.
20. Simpkins, *Long Goodnight*, 141, 145.
21. Shenk, *Forgetting*, 258.
22. Killick, "Dementia, Identity," 61.
23. Swinton, *Dementia*, 205–10.

proaches the question of identity theologically, arguing that, in contrast, God's memory of us is reliable—God knows us intimately, as we actually are across our whole lifespan, and God remembers us—and our identity is reliably held in the memory of God.[24] He presents the case that it is in God's memory that we are sustained, as God's remembering is an ongoing active remembering of us that ensures our true identity in relationship with God, now and into eternity.[25] The implications of this are significant for the church, "the only community that exists solely to bear active witness to the living memory of Jesus,"[26] that is called to be the active, embodied witness to God's remembering, reconciling, and sustaining power through the work of the Holy Spirit in the church and in the world.[27] This raises the question of how well the church, in its dealings with those whose memories need support, reflects the sustaining, reconciling, remembering God who holds the identity of each of us.

Embodied Persons

Gerontological research challenges the common assumption that cognitive impairment implies a loss of the self. On the basis of ethnographic research involving persons with dementia, Kontos argues that selfhood is articulated through social and existential aspects of the body such as gestures, appearance, social etiquette, and caring; and this embodied selfhood exists with observable coherence in bodily movements and in the capacity for caring and creativity, even into advanced dementia.[28] She argues, further, that because the self is enacted in bodily movements below the threshold of the cognitive, because it is in fact *grounded* in the corporeal, the concept of selfhood needs to be disentangled from the merely cognitive.[29] Swinton argues that the body is prior to the self and cannot be separated from it. Therefore, the actions of the body, the gestures and expressions, express meanings and memories that are manifestations of a person's subjectivity,

---

24. Ibid., 210-13. See pp. 202-26 for the extended elaboration of "living in the memories of God."
25. Ibid., 218-19.
26. Ibid., 222-23.
27. This subject is addressed in chapter 7.
28. Kontos, "Selfhood, Embodiment," 830-33.
29. Ibid., 833-35.

and so they need to be understood.[30] That the body remains an active agent has significant implications for *how* we relate and maintain mutuality in relationships *throughout* the journey of memory deterioration. A person's body language, gestures, and facial expressions call for our closest attention and respect, for a positive expectation of meaningful communication and connection. We call forth or quash the person's very self by our own embodied approach and response.

Theological anthropology also addresses the theme of embodied personhood. Barth articulates a standard theological reading of the human person as a psychosomatic unity, describing human beings as "wholly and simultaneously soul and body," with the Spirit unifying and holding these together as a body-soul unity.[31] He claims that the use of "I" for both bodily and non-bodily experiences indicates this unity, that "man has Spirit, and through the Spirit is the soul of his body,"[32] and that embodied persons are therefore to be respected, valued, and recognized as intrinsically capable of being for and in relation to God. Swinton underlines the significance of the understanding that "we are our bodies as we are our souls,"[33] and that as embodied souls we depend entirely on God for the continuation for our very life and breath. From this position of a contingent body-soul unity, he points out that because our bodies are the place where God meets and sustains us, our bodies matter, and caring for bodies is a crucial part of caring: our care for the whole person, the body-soul unity, is in effect our attending to God, and our failures in caring for persons are injustices done to God.[34] With this understanding of embodied personhood, it becomes self-evident that relating to persons with respect, and seeking to connect with, relate to, and be present with persons *in their bodies*, are indispensable in sustaining persons.

---

30. Swinton, *Dementia*, 243–47.
31. Barth, *Church Dogmatics*, 383.
32. Ibid., 394–95.
33. Swinton, *Dementia*, 167–68.
34. Ibid., 165–77.

Relational Care

Person-Centered Care

There are strong indications that the quality of personal relationships and the societal responses to a person have a major impact on a person's well-being throughout the dementia journey. Kitwood advocates practices of care where personhood is sustained in meaningful relationships, arguing that the quality of relational care is a crucial variable in the experience of dementia.[35] He spells out that for persons with dementia there is a cluster of needs—comfort, attachment, inclusion, occupation, and identity—that must be met for the *basic need for love* to be satisfied, and for personhood to be maintained. He explains that comfort is needed, especially in loss and partings, that the need for occupation can be met by projects or creative play, that identity can be fostered through continuity with the past and a narrative supported by others, and that the need for inclusion must be met, or the person will retreat and decline.[36] If these needs are met, if genuine "I-Thou" love is offered, persons with dementia may be able to move out of grief, anger, and fear, and into a more tranquil acceptance of life and death.[37]

Supportive Care

Two decades on from Kitwood's new paradigm, the goals of much supportive dementia care are to affirm the person's personhood, to strive for the person's emotional well-being, and to acknowledge the person's social value. However, attitudes that undermine a sense of personhood—such as negative stereotyping, negative self-stereotyping, and malignant social positioning of persons with dementia—are found to be still commonplace, and come into play immediately from diagnosis on.[38] Baldwin expresses concern also about a tendency to veer away from Kitwood's original concept of subject-to-subject relational care towards care that is done *to* the person, with "care management" that seeks, by means of various interventions across the system, to maintain and retrieve "the person behind the

---

35. Kitwood, *Dementia Reconsidered*, 80–84.
36. Ibid., 84–85.
37. Ibid., 10–12.
38. Sabat, "Maintaining Self," 227–31.

dementia."³⁹ Rather than such a systems approach, Baldwin advocates a "life-world" approach—undergirded by a dynamic concept of personhood that is relational at its core—that values the *present* person in this person's uniqueness, in terms of relationality.⁴⁰ Acknowledging the value of Kitwood's approach of "I-Thou" rather than "I-It" relationships, Baldwin proposes care that supports physical, psychological, and spiritual wholeness in mutual and interdependent "I-Thou" relationships, and consequently promotes the life and health of a society.⁴¹

Dementia research on the "self" endorses the view that it is the capacity for relationship that is central in sustaining the identity of persons. Exploring interpersonal dynamics from a social constructivist perspective, Sabat distinguishes three different selves: the self of personal identity (Self 1), the self as a totality of attributes (Self 2), and the socially constructed self (Self 3).⁴² Sabat elaborates that Self 1—including the personal identity built up through the continuous life story and expressed through a uniquely embodied "I" with a continuous point of view—remains intact through dementia. He highlights the importance of relationship for the maintenance of Self 2, the sum of one's mental, psychological, and physical attributes, some of which endure and some of which are vulnerable to change according to the responses of others; and he argues that Self 3, made up of the variety of selves jointly constructed, displayed, and maintained in various social situations, is *entirely* dependent on the cooperation of others for its healthy existence, being sustained only if those in relationship refuse to focus on dysfunction.⁴³

Malignant social positioning and demeaning social responses are still too often the experience of persons with dementia from diagnosis onward; and contribute to the negative self-positioning of the person.⁴⁴ Sabat underlines the importance of continuing to affirm the person's positive characteristics, arguing that if other people focus on the cognitive and physical losses of Self 2, the person has no opportunity to build a healthy social self.⁴⁵ Swinton, too, notes the fragility of Self 2 in the face of malignant

39. Baldwin, "Personhood, Personalism," 188.
40. Ibid., 190.
41. Ibid., 190–95.
42. Sabat, "Selfhood," 90–94.
43. Sabat, "Maintaining Self," 231–33.
44. Ibid., 229.
45. Ibid., 229–31.

social positioning and others' negative expectations, and he elaborates the argument that Self 2 remains through dementia, held in the memory of others and supported by their narrative of the person.[46] Bender further extends the concept of Self 2, the narrative self, as a multi-dimensional self with beliefs, attitudes, goals, skills, emotions, values; and posits that the *context*—including time, space, and emotional meaning—determines the person's response and ultimately *who the person is*.[47] These perspectives emphasize the need to create environments for relational care where *whole persons* are accorded dignity, where they are supported in maintaining their selfhood, where their personal identity is recognized as continuous, where their longstanding attributes and narrative self are valued, where their emotions are acknowledged, and where they are encouraged in social interactions. The outworking of such an approach is that the social personae not only of persons with dementia, but also of those giving care, are nurtured.[48]

Context and Care

A relational care approach must therefore seek to develop an encompassing environment supportive of the person's personhood and identity. Such an approach will include support for family relationships, building care partnerships, and working for systemic change. Recent developments in supportive care build on a concept of care that goes beyond individuals caring for individuals, to care within a team of people whose values and objectives are aligned.[49] In recognition of the importance of relationships in dementia, practical measures have been taken to establish support groups where couples are encouraged to listen to one another and to explore what the experience of dementia means to each person. Such groups have produced very positive outcomes, decreasing the sense of isolation and increasing the sense of empowerment through sharing and mutual support.[50] In such ways, the personhood and relationships of persons with dementia and their caregivers are nurtured. Thus, supportive care seeks to affirm caregivers' strengths, works with persons with dementia amidst the changes, often

---

46. Swinton, *Dementia*, 95–96.
47. Bender, *Explorations*, 256–58.
48. Ibid., 223.
49. See, for example, Hughes et al., "Ingredients and Issues," 99–104.
50. Sheard, "Relationships," 22–24.

Grounding Care: Sustaining Persons in Context

over a long period, and facilitates positive relationships in the dementia journey.

Communicative Care

One of the more distressing misconceptions of negative stereotyping is reflected in the commonly voiced question, "Can you still communicate with her/him?" Certainly, there are significant challenges in communicating with persons as words become less accessible, but of course we *are* communicating with a person, in *how* (or whether) we are present to the person. As a person's verbal skills are gradually lost, other aspects of communication are still available, indeed crucial, in developing and maintaining relationship. Effective communication seeks to hear, to understand, and to connect; and such communication is vital in sustaining persons whose verbal skills are vulnerable to change.[51] We can employ skills of connecting: through our physical positioning in relation to the person; through our body language, eye contact, tone of voice, interpreting, mirroring, being silent; and through our being really present with the person "in the moment."[52] Along with these skills, effective communication will arise from looking for a person's strengths, from a *desire* to connect person to person, from an expectant attitude that assumes that communication is possible—indeed, from our ongoing, active, expectant, listening presence.

Engagement in meaningful communication raises important questions. There is no evidence that persons with dementia lose the capacity to experience emotions; indeed, evidence suggests that they are possibly *more* emotionally attuned as their cognitive resources diminish.[53] There may be concern as to whether, through effective communication, persons with dementia will be led into grief and pain that is overwhelming and beyond their ability to process; on the other hand, there is a distinct possibility that any assumptions on our part of their emotional unawareness of their losses might be *our* way of coping with the pain, and we must ask whether anyone else has a right to seek to protect them from their own feelings of grief.[54] If we believe that our own emotions should be allowed appropriate expression and acknowledgment, we surely have no right to deny any persons

---

51. Allan and Killick, "Communicating," 218.
52. Ibid., 222–24.
53. Killick and Allan, *Communication*, 305.
54. Ibid., 306.

such expression and validation. These are important considerations, for if we fail to recognize that persons with dementia have the same emotions, hopes, and needs as others, if we fail to respect and listen to them, we create barriers to their finding meaning, hope, and connection;[55] and we depersonalize both them and ourselves.

Empathic Care

Effective communication and relational engagement call for empathy, whereby we seek to enter into and understand the world of the other as fully as possible, given our own limitations in understanding and the limitations of the other in self-understanding.[56] Pembroke explains that such participation in the other person's world is an active process whereby, in the imagination, one enters into the thinking and feeling of the other. Such imaginative projection on the part of a therapist (or listener) has the dual role of reducing a person's sense of existential aloneness and facilitating identity-building. Through telling one's story and being heard well in relationship, one is able both to discover and to draw together identity fragments into a stronger "I."[57] Effective communication and empathy play a vital role then in sustaining persons—those who are forgetting and those who accompany them—through participating in their emotional world and facilitating the rebuilding of the sense of self throughout the dementia journey.

Narrative Supportive Care

Narrative is increasingly being linked with developing and sustaining the sense of self. Baldwin draws our attention to the power of narrative in constituting and understanding ourselves and organizing our understandings of one another, and he promotes "narrative supportive care" for persons with dementia.[58] This power of narrative, he argues, facilitates the building of an inclusive overarching narrative by means of which the physical, emotional, psychological, social, and spiritual dimensions of the person are nurtured

---

55. MacKinlay and Trevitt, *Spiritual Reminiscence*, 156.
56. Pembroke, *Renewing Practice*, 72.
57. Ibid., 73–77.
58. Baldwin, "Narrative, Supportive Care," 245–46.

throughout the dementia journey.[59] He points out that meta-narratives such as a medical model of dementia—with a focus on cognitive decline and treatment of the person with dementia as a care *recipient*—can distort the narrative web; and he advocates a positive meta-narrative of hope, inspiration, and comfort, rather than of loss and decline.[60] Within such a positive framework, if both the person with dementia and the family are active agents in weaving together the web of narratives (past, present, and future), a sense of continuity with the past will be maintained, and each person will be supported in the sense of self and empowered for the journey.[61]

A narrative approach used in pastoral counseling recognizes the value of narrative in empowering persons to discover and constitute themselves. In building a positive counter-story that speaks more loudly than the current negative story, a distressed person may be encouraged to identify and reflect on "sparkling moments," unique positive outcomes in the person's present challenges or in the past, which are elaborated and incorporated into the counter-story.[62] Beyond the pastoral relationship, a "nurturing third"—a support person or supportive community—participates in this pastoral process, affirming and encouraging the positives, and sharing in building a life-sustaining counter-story.[63]

In light of a major study facilitating spiritual reminiscence with persons with dementia, MacKinlay and Trevitt emphasize the value of narrative in finding meaning and moving toward gero-transcendence and final life-meaning.[64] In this study, the sharing of reminiscence in groups acknowledged and fostered a sense of worth, and facilitated connection on a spiritual level.[65] The authors, and the narratives they report, remind us that we must not assume that difficulties in articulating the story indicate either an absence of story or loss of identity; it may take time and attentiveness, but as the story is articulated meaning is found.[66] The added benefit of group reminiscence is the empathy and mutual support offered by persons with dementia to one another. As this reminiscence work illustrates, with

---

59. Ibid., 246–48.
60. Ibid., 249–51.
61. Ibid., 250–51.
62. Pembroke, *Renewing Practice*, 63.
63. Ibid., 64–65.
64. MacKinlay and Trevitt, *Spiritual Reminiscence*, 86–90.
65. Ibid., 27–29.
66. Ibid., 16–18.

opportunities for sharing narrative through effective listening, relationships are enhanced, grief is shared, meaning is made, losses are transcended, and the story can be told powerfully. The authors argue that if persons with dementia share their story with a pastoral caregiver through the journey, meaning might be found and hope strengthened.[67]

The Caregiver

Caregiver Challenges

While the relational context is of great significance for the quality of life of a person with dementia, the impacts of caregiving on family caregivers are multiple. The demands placed on them are well-known. These include the provision of physical care and increased supervision of the person with dementia, decision-making, financial and care management, and the provision of emotional support, in the midst of significant changes in behavior, personality, and relationship. Caregivers' quality of life deteriorates, with less time for self and other family members, a loss of outside interests and contact with other people, increased family conflict, a financial toll, chronic exhaustion, health challenges, and emotional impacts such as stress and loneliness.[68] Initially denial, fear of dementia, and stoicism may deter caregiving partners from seeking help,[69] and later, particularly if the social network has failed or been withdrawn, it may seem too late.

The challenges for caregivers do not necessarily diminish if the loved one is placed in residential care. Australian research found that the decision to place the loved one in permanent care was accompanied by high stress and relentless grief; and the person's move introduced a new stressful situation for the caregiver, at least as difficult as caregiving at home.[70] Caregivers' emotional challenges at this stage of caring included loss, guilt, intense grief and a sense of meaninglessness in their separation from the loved one, concern about the person's well-being, and adjustment to a different caring role. At this time, caregivers longed for support in processing their changes in role, their loss of control of caregiving, and their loss of relationship.[71]

---

67. Ibid., 164–67.
68. Goldsmith, *Strange Land*, 100–101.
69. Bramble et al., "Seeking Connection," 3121.
70. Moyle et al., "Living with Loss," 28–29.
71. Ibid., 30.

(Of course, the other half of this picture of relocation is its impact on the person being relocated, often at a time when grief can no longer be verbally processed, where connection with the caregiver and familiarity with the home environment are desperately clung to for security, and where confusion and a sense of abandonment may already prevail.) A caregiver's grief at the time of and following the loved one's death presents further huge challenges.[72] These ongoing challenges and their emotional costs to caregivers obviously affect not only themselves but also the environment and the well-being of persons with dementia. Such demands raise the question of what constitutes appropriate spiritual/pastoral care for caregivers, on the journey as a whole and in each of the most difficult periods of adjustment.

A Pastoral Challenge

These perspectives, then, offer a foundational understanding of God-given and inviolable personhood, and of persons as embodied, emotional, spiritual, relational beings. With this starting point comes the serious responsibility of sustaining and nurturing the whole person, in *every* aspect. The sociological recognition of the importance of relationship and social context finds resounding support in the theological understanding of a relational *person*, sustained in loving relationship with God and others. The concept of the self as enduring personal identity, attributes, and social personae throws valuable light on how to acknowledge the loss of cognitive and physical attributes while still affirming the present person and sustaining this person in relationship.

Acknowledging the centrality of relationships, theological perspectives support much of the current social scientific dementia research and its outworking in relational person-centered, person-honoring care practices. In emphasizing the value of the whole person—the body-spirit unity, which includes the vertical dimension of relationship with God, who created human beings for relationship—such understandings challenge any care that ignores the spiritual dimension and the interrelatedness of all dimensions of human life. On the other hand, any approach to pastoral care that addresses the "spiritual" as an entity *apart from* the other aspects of a person's life is cause for grave concern. The serious attention given in cultural research to developing best practice in person-centered, relational,

---

72. Grief is discussed in chapter 5.

and supportive care presents a challenge to the Christian community concerning best practice in pastoral care.

We have the theological understanding of personhood bestowed by God on persons created in God's image, created for loving relationship. Let us reflect on Anderson's challenge that our abstract obligation is worked out in our concrete encounter with persons, and that our withholding what is necessary for the well-being of another person's embodied, personal existence denies our own participation in God's love.[73] Indeed, such withholding throws into question our very humanity; as Barth argues, our humanness consists in seeing, speaking with, listening to, assisting and being assisted by other persons, and being with our fellow human beings gladly.[74]

So we face the responsibility, as individuals and as Christian community, not to withhold what others need, but to respond with the relational, overflowing love of the triune God to persons on the dementia journey—both those who are forgetting and those who accompany them—whose personhood, like our own, is sustained in relationship with God and other people. As we reflect on the moral and theological challenge to respond appropriately, and as we learn from current cultural understandings and their potential for supportive care, we come to the pastoral challenge of sustaining persons in the midst of the losses that dementia brings; and we continue to explore the means by which we can respond gladly.

---

73. Anderson, *Being Human*, 74.
74. Barth, *Church Dogmatics*, 264–84.

2

Grounding Pastoral Care: Spirituality and Meaning

Scientific medicine may be able to provide us the means to live longer and healthier lives, but it is utterly powerless to offer us any meaning to live for. But that is precisely what spiritual care does offer, and therefore, why it is so crucial in supportive dementia care.
—Stephen Sapp, "Spiritual Care"

Spirituality

Scope and Meanings

WITH THE UNDERSTANDING THAT we are personal, embodied, relational, and spiritual beings, to what are we referring when we speak of spirituality and spiritual care? Current conceptualizations of spirituality range widely: from the personal search for meaning and connection with the transcendent[1] to what *gives* continuing meaning and purpose and nourishes the inner being;[2] from a "quest for meaning, purpose, self-transcending knowledge, meaningful relationships, love, and commitment, as well as the sense of the Holy amongst us,"[3] to a human spirituality that seeks an answer totally within oneself to the question "How do you make sense out of a world

---

1. MacKinlay and Trevitt, *Spiritual Reminiscence*, 18.
2. Jewell, "Nourishing the Spirit," 14–16.
3. Swinton and Mowat, *Practical Theology*, 238.

that does not seem to be intrinsically reasonable?"[4] These definitions reflect something of the breadth of the spectrum, from the search within to the relational, outward, upward quest for the transcendent, and from inner nourishment to intentional living in relation to a Higher Power. In fact, it may be argued that spirituality is so integral to being human that it defies the boundaries of definition; nonetheless, the range of definitions offers common ground in the search for meaning, connection, and transcendence.

The terms "spirituality" and "religion" are now often differentiated; and although there are wide-ranging views on how they differ, some commonality exists. McCarthy, adopting a theological perspective, argues that spirituality precedes and is more encompassing than any formal religious system, but when the universal quest for meaning involves reference to God or the Divine, it becomes religious.[5] From a psychological perspective, it is argued that spirituality may be seen as the broader construct, while the religious search for the sacred "unfolds within a traditional sacred context"[6] or faith tradition, with embedded values, practices, and beliefs.[7] In seeking to clarify the bounds of spirituality and religion, Jewell's model is helpful. This model depicts concentric circles, from an inclusive circle of universal human spirituality (intangible, sustaining qualities and values), to a second circle within that represents the spirituality of different faith traditions, to an inner circle of Christian spirituality, and, central to the model, the circle of an individual person's spirituality.[8]

While it is the intrinsic, personal aspects of religion or spirituality that are often the focus, the importance of tradition and context for religion cannot be underestimated. Authentic religious spirituality is usually expressed through participation in a faith community held together by common beliefs, practices, and values.[9] To what extent one's religion is practiced in community is obviously relevant to how a person's self-identity is sustained, how trials are faced, and from whom assistance is sought.[10] Older people may call on their religion in orienting themselves in the changing circumstances and uncertain experiences of ageing; and they may turn to their

---

4. Morgan, "Existential Quest," 6.
5. McCarthy, "Spirituality," 196–97.
6. Zinnbauer and Pargament, "Religiousness," 35.
7. Ibid., 33–37.
8. Jewell, "Nourishing the Spirit," 22–24.
9. McCarthy, "Spirituality," 197–200.
10. Park and Paloutzian, "Integration," 554–56.

religious social environment for opportunities to explore questions of life's meaning and value with others.[11] In a stressful situation, people may seek support from other members of their church community and the clergy, and may receive meaningful support and a sense of being cared for within the religious support network; on the other hand, crisis may bring confusion and disappointment about these spiritual network relationships, if latent expectations of support are not met.[12] Thus, coping in difficult life circumstances may be assisted by a person's religion, depending on its form, its application, and the quality of support within the religious community.

A search for meaning, then, is generally identified as an important aspect of spirituality and in particular of spirituality in aging. Older people inevitably face loss, including a loss of earlier purposes and goals; and, very possibly, they may experience loneliness and pain. Questions of life's meaning may surface and become more pressing. Coping and resilience are associated with the tasks of transcending loss, and moving towards wholeness and peace within oneself and in relation to others, and towards ultimate life meaning and spiritual integrity.[13]

A person makes meaning and interprets and assimilates changes within a framework of global meaning that includes the person's beliefs, subjective feelings, goals, and sense of purpose in life.[14] Within a framework of global meaning, the person's identity is constructed and reconstructed in interaction with others across a lifetime, and one's personal narrative may be developed in a wider religious narrative.[15] This framework is the context for structures of meaning within which we assimilate change and interpret events; however, there are some events and associated losses that disrupt one's set of values and challenge one's assumptive world.[16] Where established value systems are inadequate to handle the new demands, the task of coping calls for a new set of goals or purpose.[17] Difficult life challenges such as crisis, suffering, loss, and a loved one's death may produce incongruence between the global and situational meaning, and usher in

---

11. Eisenhandler, *Keeping Faith*, 19.
12. Pargament et al., "Coping," 483–86.
13. MacKinlay and Trevitt, *Spiritual Reminiscence*, 86–90.
14. Park, "Religion and Meaning," 297.
15. Ozorak, "Cognitive Approaches," 226–28.
16. Marris, "Holding onto Meaning," 14–18.
17. Pargament, *Religion and Coping*, 239.

a meaning-making process to reduce stress and facilitate adjustment.[18] In order to recover, one may need to adjust goals, reinterpret the present situation to fit within the assumptive world, or—if established value systems are inadequate to handle the new demands—one's long held beliefs and values may be rejected.[19]

Negative or distressing events may be appraised more positively through the lens of faith, and people within a religious framework have been found to engage more readily than others in cognitive processing.[20] Suffering may be interpreted as part of an overall benevolent plan of God, or as an opportunity for spiritual growth and learning; and such appraisals may bring comfort and meaning.[21] On the other hand, where God is blamed there may be anger that leads to depression and poor coping skills, and possibly doubt and rejection of belief.[22] In such situations, the experiential aspect of a person's suffering needs to be addressed, for example through normalizing a sense of distance from God and facilitating the expression of negative feelings to God; and when the feelings are validated and normalized, a person may be more able to appraise the situation positively.[23]

In critical or demanding circumstances, there may be spiritual distress, involving a sense of disconnection within oneself, or conflict between one's interpretation of the circumstances and one's global meaning, or a disruption of one's social connections. There may be feelings of vulnerability, an overwhelming loneliness, or a void that challenges one's ability to derive any meaning from existence.[24] Such existential disconnectedness and meaninglessness become all-encompassing and beyond the emotional realm;[25] they are spiritual issues, and must therefore be addressed at a spiritual level. Spiritual distress or pain in such demanding circumstances calls for empathy, compassion, humanity, and at times silent presence, in a spiritual environment where people are encouraged to connect with their own spiritual resources within their own belief system and network.[26] Through

---

18. Park, "Religion and Meaning," 304–7.
19. Ibid., 307–8.
20. Pargament et al., "Coping," 481.
21. Ibid., 482–84.
22. Exline and Rose "Spiritual Struggles," 317–19.
23. Ibid., 321–24.
24. McGrath, "Spiritual Pain," 639–45.
25. Speck, "Spiritual Care," 251–53.
26. Mitchell et al., "Spiritual Distress," 366–69.

such connection, with its opportunities for meaning-making, spiritual distress may not ultimately be negative but rather may offer the possibility of rebuilding and growth.

Crises and challenges to one's assumptive world are difficult to confront alone, and yet the loss of significant relationships is a stark reality in aging. Whether people are able to access support in the challenges is a pertinent question. Coleman argues that where aging people face either crises of meaning in their individual lives or questions of life's meaning in general, religion is a traditional bulwark; and where there is a decline in religious belonging, health and well-being are threatened.[27] He notes the dearth of opportunities for older people to discuss issues of faith, values, and meaning; and he observes that churches, while often employing ministry agents for younger cohorts, seldom do so for the elderly.[28] Susan and John McFadden reflect on older people's experience of becoming increasingly "invisible" in congregations, and then in their late years, experiencing the condescension of others; and they make the point that in faith communities in particular, all persons in all circumstances should be honored.[29]

Spiritual Care

In light of these current understandings of spirituality and spiritual issues, what is the place of spiritual caregiving, and to whom and how should it be provided? Anderson argues from a theological perspective that human beings are spiritual, social, and physical, all three interconnected spheres being essential to the person's selfhood; and therefore all authentic caregiving is spiritual.[30] Spiritual well-being is identified with love, meaning and purpose, hope, joy, creativity, and peace, whereas ill-being is characterized by isolation, despair, sadness, boredom, and anxiety.[31] As spiritual needs are core human needs, spiritual care focuses on nurturing wellness and well-being in the midst of challenges, and addresses a wide range of issues and tasks. Such tasks include exploring existential questions of meaning in life and suffering; nurturing communication, relationship, and peace; validating the emotions and offering comfort; encouraging the giving and

27. Coleman "Ageing and Personhood," 65–68.
28. Ibid., 67.
29. McFadden and McFadden, *Aging Together*, 135–36.
30. Anderson, *Spiritual Caregiving*, 9–10.
31. Jewell, "Nourishing the Spirit," 23.

receiving of love and forgiveness; facilitating creative activities and play; fostering meaning and purpose; and engaging with a person in the journey toward transcendence.

There are calls for an interdisciplinary team model of community support that includes spiritual care: to support aging and facilitate meaning-making as a spiritual journey,[32] to support spiritual practices and faith-based coping, and to nurture the spirituality of people in the community and in aged care centers, regardless of whether or not they are religious.[33] Swinton warns that a narrow understanding of spirituality may marginalize and exclude some groups, including those with cognitive impairment.[34] This warning is timely in a hyper-cognitive culture where there may be assumptions that spirituality relates to the power to think and to be self-directed, a view implicit in such comments as: "the first degree of spirituality is knowledge,"[35] and the "ability of persons to self-determine his or her life is perhaps the most fundamental example of the spiritual nature of the person."[36] Where persons with dementia are at risk of being denied their spirituality, we need to stand against such marginalization.

Spiritual Care in the Dementia Journey

Could it be that enabling people to function within the spiritual dimension is in fact a key which can unlock the person and reveal dimensions of personhood that appear lost until they are encountered in the stillness of that spiritual moment?
—JOHN SWINTON, "BEING IN THE MOMENT"

In many ways, the spiritual care offered to persons with dementia should be no different from that offered to anyone else, as persons with memory loss are *not* in some different category that sets them apart; the needs are the same human needs for love, relationship, connection, hope, comfort, creativity, and transcendence that have been discussed. Nonetheless, in the dementia journey there are particular opportunities and challenges

---

32. Mowat, "Ageing," 118–20.
33. Goldsmith, "Spirituality and Non-religious," 170–72.
34. Swinton, *Mental Health Care*, 24.
35. Morgan, "Existential Quest," 7.
36. Ibid., 8.

that demand sensitivity and understanding, and offer significant—indeed key—possibilities for sustaining persons.

Spiritual Care and Persons with Dementia

Relationships and Connection

As is the case with any spiritual care, relationships are fundamentally important in spiritual care for persons with dementia. In early dementia, there may be feelings of loss, isolation, fear, and worthlessness; and spiritual care must seek ways of addressing these challenges and bringing healing to the sense of disconnection that comes with memory loss. In promoting spiritual well-being, spiritual care must emerge out of reciprocal relationships offered by care *partners*—it is not *something done to* a person.[37] Meaningful relationships involve giving and receiving love, and sharing joy and sorrow; and thus they do not require an intellectual component.[38] While reciprocity is not always guaranteed, we can grow in our understanding of ourselves and our own selfhood as we share time and friendship in affirming and sustaining the selfhood of another.[39]

Relationship-building with persons with dementia requires sensitivity and skill in communicating. An *expectation* of connection is fundamental to such communication—many who relate to persons with dementia have noted their intuitive discernment of what is genuine and what is not. Mowat offers a framework for accessing the spiritual domain through relationship-building; and she argues for a creative, expressive space, wherein relationships are developed through employing both verbal and non-verbal communication with persons in *their* reality, and where sustained spiritual conversations and storytelling can facilitate connection and hope.[40]

Various research studies have sought to listen to and explore the spiritual experience of persons with dementia themselves. Snyder, after hearing the stories of many persons with dementia, underlines the need for compassionate listening that acknowledges the grief of losses fundamental to a person's "very sense of self."[41] In qualitative research into the satisfactions

---

37. MacKinlay, "Creating Care," 45–46.
38. McFadden and McFadden, *Aging Together*, 59–61.
39. Ibid., 77–82.
40. Mowat, "Voicing the Spiritual," 78–84.
41. Snyder, *Speaking Our Minds*, 51.

and challenges of spirituality for persons with dementia, Snyder found that spirituality and religion were rich resources for finding meaning, connection, and sustenance; and she makes the point that early in dementia people may need to discuss challenges to faith such as diminishing cognition, the meaning in the situation, and meaning for the rest of life, and later in the journey to explore fears about relationship with God and loss of peace.[42] Through her listening to many persons with dementia, Kotai-Ewers found that while each person's expression of spirituality was unique, there was also a commonality in seeking meaning, and a need for persons to talk to find meaning in the experience and in life; and she found a common awareness of loss, death, and a spiritual dimension.[43] A major study with persons with dementia who participated in small spiritual reminiscence groups revealed that, along with the articulation of spiritual memories and present faith, the groups facilitated the processing of grief and a meaning-making process that might otherwise be blocked.[44] The conversations revealed hopes and needs similar to those of other people, but also indicated that there were specific barriers to hope in the attitudes of others and in the failure of others to listen.[45] Such sharing of stories, within a relationship of trust, may lead to the discovery and acceptance of meaning in the diagnosis, and may thus open the way to hope and well-being.[46]

Identity

As has been discussed, the dementia journey challenges a person's sense of identity and may bring a sense of disconnection from the self; and finding ways of maintaining continuity with the self and with the past is important in nurturing the person's identity. A foundational tool in relationship-building is empathy, whereby the pain of aloneness is eased as the listener enters the person's world, and through being heard well, the person is empowered to build a stronger sense of identity.[47] Swinton notes that "presence is remembrance in action," and the person's identity is held well by

---

42. Snyder, "Satisfactions and Challenges," 306–7.
43. Kotai-Ewers, *Listen*, 135–37.
44. MacKinlay and Trevitt, *Spiritual Reminiscence*, 185.
45. Ibid., 156–57.
46. MacKinlay, "Creating Care," 43–44.
47. Mowat, "Voicing the Spiritual," 72–78.

companions who listen "with eyes, ears and soul."[48] Connecting persons with their past not only acknowledges their accomplishments and identity, but facilitates the rediscovery of what earlier spiritual or religious resources have sustained them in difficult times; and thus their current well-being is supported.[49] The means of connecting with the past include memory cueing through the senses, natural beauty, and music,[50] and life review and memory boxes.[51]

The experience of one person dealing with the question of identity in dementia offers insight into spiritual possibilities in the midst of identity challenges. Early in her journey, Christine Bryden experiences the fear of the "loss of self."[52] Later in the journey, however, she writes:

> As my cognition fades, my spirituality can flourish as an important source of identity. As I lose an identity in the world around me, which is so anxious to define me by what I do and say, . . . I can seek an identity by simply being me, a person created in the image of God.[53]

Later again, and still with a forward-looking perspective, Bryden reflects on the importance of ongoing spiritual growth in sustaining her identity amid the losses: "by focusing on my spirit in relationship with the divine, I am becoming who I really am."[54] In her amazing journey in dementia, two decades after her diagnosis, this remarkable person writes:

> The meaning of my life is to be in relationship with Jesus, and this may well become even stronger for me as the masks of cognition and emotion fall away further to reveal my inner spirit. Many people with dementia may find themselves profoundly spiritual as they journey closer to death . . . so it's crucial they're not excluded from their spiritual practices.[55]

---

48. Swinton, *Dementia*, 239.
49. Shamy, *Spiritual Dimension*, 76–77.
50. Ibid., 77–81.
51. Goldsmith, *Strange Land*, 94–96.
52. Boden, *Who Will I Be?* 48.
53. Bryden and MacKinlay, "Spiritual Journey," 71.
54. Bryden, *Dancing with Dementia*, 158.
55. Bryden, *Before I Forget*, 273.

Spiritual Connection

Such insights underline the importance of nurturing the relational, emotional, and spiritual life of persons on this journey. As in other relationships, pastoral or personal, a positive, trusting, accepting attitude facilitates connection and spiritual encounter; and in getting to know and love a person with dementia deeply, "soul-to-soul connection" may occur in silence and presence.[56] Drawing on the contemplative tradition with its practice of stillness, presence, and sacred connection, where God the Spirit is encountered in the openness and expectancy of the moment, Swinton points to the possibilities of deep connection with a person into severe dementia, in a space where each moment is a sacrament filled with new possibilities and hope.[57] Killick, who has spent much time in listening, describes interactions that indicate deep interconnectedness and spiritual connection with persons with minimal language.[58] Thus time, presence, and silence are gifts with immeasurable potential for establishing and maintaining relational, spiritual connection and so nurturing persons—those who give the gift of presence as well as those who receive it, as they share together in the presence of the Spirit.

Worship

For those for whom particular faith practices are familiar, these practices support the continuity of identity in the dementia journey. There is ample anecdotal evidence that persons can still share in the core elements of worship despite significant memory loss;[59] and it is widely recognized that people's religious heritage must be valued through ensuring access to appropriate acts of worship and religious services. Worship opportunities should facilitate connection and a sense of continuity with past worship practices through familiar rituals, music, prayers.[60] Expressions of creativity are recognized as elements of spirituality, and the creative arts can be

---

56. Lenshyn, "Living Echo," 21–23.
57. Swinton, "Contemplative Approach," 184–85.
58. Killick, "Friend of Time," 58–62.
59. Schultz, *Not Forgotten*, 86.
60. For practical guidelines for appropriate and meaningful worship see Shamy, *Spiritual Dimension*, 98–115, and Schultz, *Not Forgotten*, 85–92.

employed to cater for all the senses and a "sixth sense of the transcendent."[61] Providing opportunities for creativity and play fosters the spiritual growth of those who can express themselves in these ways, and also those who are involved in offering this ministry.[62]

Sustained in Faith Communities

The role of the spiritual community in the dementia journey is increasingly being acknowledged. Memory can be seen as something "that resides in community, tradition and place, and so is not entirely dependent on any one individual's level of cognitive function,"[63] and Christian communities are called to be reservoirs of memory where the person is held in the memories of others who are attentive to the person and to the presence of God in the person.[64] Bryden challenges the Christian community to determine at what point her selfhood and spirituality are to be denied her, and suggests that it is the stigma of dementia that places limits on participation in spiritual practices.[65] The challenge to the Christian community is summed up by Everett, who spent much time ministering among persons with dementia:

> The cognitively impaired still have emotions, imagination, a will and moral awareness far into the disease process. Feelings retain importance and influence long beyond the time when they can be understood or articulated. These aspects of emotions and imagination are the vital wellsprings from which we experience life's meaning. How can we abandon these people in our ministry of God unless we have a very limited understanding of how God is experienced?[66]

The importance of an accepting, loving community for persons with dementia is put succinctly from first-hand experience: "the last thing we ever lose is love. Our memories may be gone. Intellect and logic may have

---

61. Allen, "Remembering," 13.
62. McFadden, "Creative Expression," 101–2.
63. Allen, "Sounding the Depths," 163.
64. Swinton, *Dementia*, 222–23.
65. Bryden and MacKinlay, "Spiritual Journey," 71–75.
66. Everett, "Forget Me Not," 80.

diminished. We may have forgotten your name and where we are, or what we are doing. But we remember love."[67]

In the pastoral studies field, texts that address the spiritual care of persons with dementia also acknowledge the multiple challenges faced by family caregivers. Shamy notes the practical, spiritual, and emotional challenges of caregiving, and particularly the spiritual yearning and the threatened loss of personal identity of caregivers; and from her experience as a caregiving daughter, she speaks of an absence of pastoral understanding.[68] Schultz acknowledges the spiritual search for meaning in the caregiving experience, along with guilt, anxiety, isolation, anger, and sadness.[69] In written narratives of caregivers, a picture emerges of grief and a longing for that grief to be acknowledged pastorally. Allford expresses disappointment at the inadequacy of pastoral ministry from the church where her parents had been active for many years, not only for her mother with dementia but also for the family, and for her father in his deep grief.[70] Among the emotional and spiritual challenges of a caregiver's journey, grief claims its place.

The Challenge to Care

In summary, historically, care for persons with dementia focused on their medical condition rather than on whole persons in their whole context. With a paradigm shift in the past two to three decades in the human sciences, support for persons with dementia through appropriate care has assumed increasing importance. There is acknowledgment of each person's status as a relational human being, increasingly dependent on those providing care for their personhood to be nurtured and their well-being to be guaranteed; and great strides have been made in the development of person-centered, relational, communicative, supportive care within a supportive environment. A person's spirituality, including meaning-making and connection with the self, others, and the transcendent, is recognized as having a contribution to well-being. Spiritual resources and a supportive spiritual community have the potential to support and foster coping; but where there is disappointment about a lack of support, and difficulties in meaning-making and in reconciling the present situation with the person's

67. Brennan, "Message of Love," 6.
68. Shamy, *Spiritual Dimension*, 63–70.
69. Schultz, *Not Forgotten*, 67–69.
70. Allford, "Relative's Perspective," 24–26.

assumptive world, there may be negative outcomes. Spiritual distress may accompany crisis and significant loss; and calls for spiritual care to be a component of a multidisciplinary response in the provision of care should be heard.

Theologically, we begin with a person created in the image of God and therefore ontologically constituted as a relational body-spirit unity, sustained as a whole person in loving relationship with God and other people. To nurture persons on the dementia journey, the context and relationships must be supportive of their personhood, their identity, and their emotional and spiritual journey; and those who accompany and care for the person must, themselves, be sustained physically, emotionally, relationally, and spiritually. These themes and insights from cultural and pastoral sources offer principles, pointers, and practices to be heeded if persons on the dementia journey are to be sustained. To listen is central to pastoral practice, and we now turn to hear the experience of the journey as described by individual caregivers.

3

Caregiving: A Lived Experience

Descriptions and Meanings: Interpretive Phenomenological Research

IN DEVELOPING A COMPREHENSIVE approach to pastoral care, it is important to hear the voices of those traveling the journey and to explore their stories. While there have been recent studies, both qualitative and quantitative, addressing particular aspects of caregivers' experience of caring, little research has explored caregivers' perceptions of the ongoing impacts of the dementia journey on their emotions and spirituality, or of the impacts of their spirituality on the experience, or of what would constitute emotional and spiritual support. We direct our attention toward these ends through a qualitative study of the caregiving journey.

Interpretive Phenomenological Analysis: Methodology

To better understand the experience of the journey, an Interpretive Phenomenological Analysis approach is employed. Having its roots in psychology, this is a method of describing, exploring, and analyzing the experiences and perspectives articulated by a small number of individuals, in order to gain deeper understanding of a specific situation or phenomenon.[1] The approach is gaining popularity in health studies and is adaptable

---

1. Pringle et al., "Interpretive Phenomenological Analysis," 20.

to other fields where the intention is to hear and understand the needs of those whose experience differs from the usual, with a view to improving support services.[2] The analysis is intensive and detailed—made possible because of the small number of participants—as it seeks to approach each person's experience on its own terms, allowing the individual experience to reveal itself as itself.[3] In seeking to hear, understand, and communicate the meaning of the experience for individuals, the researcher's interpretation is firmly grounded in participants' own words,[4] while the researcher's previous experience becomes part of the interpretive process.[5] Then, bringing together the individual experiences, the researcher seeks commonalities and divergences, and interprets the meaning of these experiences of the phenomenon in the broader context.[6]

The degree to which such a study might have general application should be considered. While it does not claim to be generalizable, an Interpretive Phenomenological study may be judged by whether it illuminates the broader context; and where there is transparency and coherence in the process, where limitations are openly acknowledged, and where the findings are related to current literature, the reader is able to assess transferability.[7] Rigor in the study is achieved through a clear auditable process of systematic analysis. Method triangulation—achieved through employing multiple methods of data collection, including recorded interviews and subsequent researcher journal entries—further enhances validity and transparency.[8] In processing the data, credibility and fittingness are achieved through member-checking, to validate the accuracy of reception and to hear whether the themes that emerge accord with participants' experience.[9]

What is sought in the initial phase is a coherent, credible description of the personal meaning of the experience, faithful to the participant's story. The process is user-friendly and non-prescriptive, with recorded conversational interviews that allow for an intimacy with the experience and the

---

2. Ibid., 21–23.
3. Larkin et al., "Giving Voice," 108.
4. Ibid., 103.
5. Pringle et al., "Interpretive Phenomenological Analysis," 22–23.
6. Ibid., 21–22.
7. Smith et al., "Interpretive Phenomenological Analysis," 51–53.
8. Ibid., 183.
9. Swinton and Mowat, *Practical Theology*, 123–25.

data.¹⁰ Immersing herself in the data, the researcher seeks central concerns, themes, and meanings for the person, dialoguing reflexively between the data, the interpretation, and field notes; and the act of writing forms the research process.¹¹ Individual accounts stand alone as important data; and the goal of the data analysis is to offer a "thick," contextualized description of participants' lived experience, and to interpret what this means to them and what it means in the wider context.¹² Then, bringing together the individual analyses, the data is analyzed for convergent and divergent experiences and themes across participants, exemplars emerging that characterize common themes across participants.¹³ The participants' stories are told, the themes and interconnections are traced, and they find their place and meaning within the broader context of knowledge and theory.

The Study

This research study, undertaken in accordance with the Human Ethics processes of the University of Queensland, engaged a sample of six caregiver participants; and in order to facilitate a deep exploration of specific, enduring, and changing issues, three interviews were conducted with each participant across a year. The participants were recruited either through a Community Care service or using a snowballing method where friends of the researcher approached caregivers known to them but unknown to the researcher, to invite participation.¹⁴ This allowed access to the "hidden population" of caregivers not receiving community support. Though the sample was small, it encompassed a quite wide range of experiences, and captured something of the challenges of long-term caregiving as well as the at times rapidly changing nature of the experience. Of the six, one had not had connection with a church, two had some connection, and three had been or were very involved in Christian congregations. Participants included caregivers whose loved one had recently been diagnosed, those further into the journey, and one after the loved one's death, where insights were shared about the present experience and retrospectively about the caring journey.

10. Pringle et al., "Interpretive Phenomenological Analysis," 21–22.
11. Crist and Tanner, "Interpretation/Analysis," 203.
12. Larkin et al., "Giving Voice," 104.
13. Ibid., 202–3.
14. Eisenhandler, *Keeping Faith*, 12–13.

Caregiving: A Lived Experience

The stories and meanings of caregiving were sought from within, where individual experiences, understandings, and perceptions were described and reflected on.[15] A conversational approach sought to capture what was important to the person, while minimizing the stress by co-constructing the interview. This allowed participants the freedom to explore their experience at their own pace and to organize their thoughts in their own way, while the interviewer aimed to "be present" rather than to direct the process. Interviews took place in a venue nominated by the caregiver, allowing for the possibility that in-home interviews would be more manageable for caregivers bound by demanding schedules, health challenges, and unpredictable circumstances. Very personal and potentially emotional experiences were thus able to be shared in a safe environment that gave context to the experience.

The interviews invited participants to reflect on the challenges of caring for a loved one with dementia, the emotions engendered, the spiritual impacts, the support received, and their coping strategies. Prompts were used toward the end of interviews if relevant areas had not been covered. Positive aspects of the journey were also sought, and the final prompt explored what emotional and spiritual support was desired. The subsequent interviews at six-monthly intervals invited caregivers to reflect on ongoing challenges and changes and their impacts during the previous six months, and on what the journey meant for them. Experiences from earlier interviews were followed up if not referred to spontaneously, to gain deeper insight across the time span. This format provided opportunity for sequential story-telling, and for exploration of the participants' emotional and spiritual responses to the experience.

Immediately following each interview, field notes were made in order to capture the researcher's rational and intuitive responses. The notes related to information, observation, description, and core words; and, in order to enhance the construction of meaning, the researcher journaled insights, emotional responses, and reflections. Each interview was transcribed verbatim, a pseudonym was assigned to the data set, and a thematic analysis was undertaken. Recognizing that each participant's experience stands on its own, the researcher sought the themes and meaning of the story of each interview, analyzing parts of the text in the light of the whole and vice versa, and moving between field notes and transcript. A written profile of each caregiver was developed, which sought to capture something of the essence of the ongoing journey and to describe the participant's experience as it

---

15. See Appendix B for interview guidelines.

was understood by the researcher. Following each interview, the transcript from the particular interview was read in the context of the participant's emerging picture, and the overall picture was further developed. Member checking by phone calls confirmed that the themes and meanings uncovered by the researcher represented the experience of the participant.

The participants' central concerns were identified, analyzed, and interpreted for what this experience might mean for them.[16] Cumulative coding of each transcript and integrative coding across transcripts were undertaken to develop a thematic account, and exemplars were identified that elucidated or expressed the essence of identified themes.[17] This process gave participants a voice, with the researcher's comments serving as a coordinating background voice.

Based on individual transcripts and thematic analyses, themes were analyzed across participants. Central themes were named, and excerpts were identified that vividly captured commonalities. These exemplars were used to introduce themes in the overall thematic analysis. As with individual thematic analyses, the overall thematic analysis was grounded in participants' statements. Consideration was given to the meaning of the overall thematic analysis in the wider context of recent research and theory around caregiving in the dementia journey, and a contextualized account was developed of what it might mean, emotionally and spiritually, to care for a family member with dementia. The study thus offered insights into the emotional and spiritual challenges, and what might constitute appropriate pastoral care for family caregivers on the dementia journey.

In presenting the following stories, names and biographical details have been changed in order to preserve the anonymity of participants. The words of participants have, however, been quoted without change.

Understanding the Lived Experience

Henri's Story

Profile

Henri is an eighty-three-year-old French-Australian gentleman who cares for his wife Marguerite. They have been married for twenty-one years.

---

16. Crist and Tanner, "Interpretation/Analysis," 203–4.
17. Ibid., 202.

Henri's health is precarious and deteriorating, and Marguerite has very recently been diagnosed with Alzheimer's Disease, after about two years of noticeable cognitive deterioration. Marguerite emigrated from Canada in later life and has no other family in Australia. Because of her inability to cope alone and her adamant refusal to consider residential aged care, Henri's deep and often repeated concern is for her future. If he should die, or even be hospitalized overnight, there is no one to care for Marguerite. Henri's adult children do not live close by, are very busy with their own lives and problems, and are not involved.

As well as the future concerns, the present challenges are pressing. Henri worries about Marguerite's safety in the home and the safety of the home, about her handling of finances, her constant spending, her sharing of her credit card information with other people, and her day-to-day behavior. Refusing to accept that she has memory problems, Marguerite resists his guidance or direction in all these areas, and Henri feels under constant pressure. While there are outings and social support for Marguerite from several friends, Henri has only one friend to whom, at times, he can talk.

Six months later all the concerns, both present and future, are more pressing. Marguerite's cognition has deteriorated, and Henri has had two weeks in hospital. Marguerite's friend cared for her during that time, but Marguerite's time away from her home has been very disorientating. Henri is very stressed by the daily demands of Marguerite's increasing need for care and supervision, and her resistance to being "controlled." In light of Henri's health problems, his concern about her future, and her continuing resistance to any suggestion of permanent residential care, a decision has been made that Marguerite will return to Canada to be cared for by her daughter. Marguerite is aware that this relocation is planned, and she alternates between being eager to go and unwilling to leave Henri. He plans to sell the home after her departure and move into a residential aged care center, where he will have people to talk to and to care for him.

Five months later, Henri is alone. Very recently, Marguerite's daughter has taken her to Canada, and Marguerite is confused and unhappy there. Henri is distressed about Marguerite's distress, and he is missing her very much, day and night. He is anxious about selling the house, which he is trying to do in order to relocate to somewhere where he will be cared for, and he is also anxious about this unknown future environment. He pictures it as being like jail. In his grief and anxiety, there is no one to talk to. He wishes he could win the lottery, because if he had the money he would fly Marguerite home tomorrow and pay for twenty-four-hour care for her.

Interpretive Analysis

DIVIDEDNESS AND TURMOIL

Henri describes himself as easy-going and sociable, and his description of his care-giving situation is punctuated with laughter, often hearty. This apparent joviality is strikingly incongruent with the content of his story, his agitated body language, and his often anxious, stressed tone of voice. This contrast reflects the inner dividedness that characterizes his experience of the journey. His anxiety about his own fragile health is greatly compounded by the implications for Marguerite's future care and life. While the future is constantly on his mind, there is turmoil, too, about the present. It appears that he is stretched and pulled this way and that, from the present to the future, from here where he is to wherever Marguerite is, from his thinking to his feelings, losing himself somewhere in the middle.

The journey is characterized by constant pressure, and Henri's load is heavy. Even when the concern about Marguerite's future is eased, and the load of caregiving is shifted, as he says, from his shoulders onto her daughter's shoulders, he still carries a burden of anxiety about the impact on Marguerite and on her daughter and family, and about his own future. Day and night across the year, there is no peace.

POWERLESSNESS AND CONFUSION

In his turmoil Henri seeks to take control of the situation and the future; and he is unable to do so. He interprets Marguerite's behavior as an unwillingness to cooperate and function normally, rather than an inability to do so. There are confusing contradictions in his appraisals, as on one hand he expects her to function, remember, and reason as she has done previously, and on the other hand he thinks of her as being like a naughty small child or a baby. He unsuccessfully attempts to control her behavior; and in her confusion and angry resistance to being controlled he tries, and at times fails, to control his own emotions. The relationship has previously been good, and the conflict and anger are unfamiliar and very distressing. Across the whole year he feels powerless, when Marguerite is with him, out shopping, or in another country. With his mind in confusion, he does not employ cognitive strategies to assist him in coping. By the end of the year he fears the time alone to think, concerned that he will completely lose control of his mind and "go cuckoo."

Ambiguity and ambivalence

The ambiguities of the journey are unsettling and disempowering to Henri; there is so much that he does not know. Marguerite's "illnesses" symbolize this ambiguity. Henri does not know—and Marguerite's doctor acknowledges the dilemma—whether Marguerite's intermittent pains are real and her intense and then forgotten health fears are founded; and he feels helpless and ambivalent about whether to take them seriously or ignore them. His inability to discern what she *cannot* and what she *will* not remember is frustrating, and her day-to-day fluctuations in functioning add to his sense of helplessness and frustration. The ambivalent emotions of anger and affection, relief and sadness, are reinforced in his narration by the bursts of laughter alternating with loud echoes of frustration and agitation when he relates snippets of conversations with Marguerite. For a man who describes himself as easy-going, the ambiguities and challenges have taken their toll.

Grief

For Henri, along with the confusion and ambiguity of Marguerite's status, loved wife or resistant child, close companion or difficult infant, there is loss and grief. However, it is difficult to accept and grieve the losses while still expecting Marguerite to behave as she did formerly. The anticipatory grief of the impending separation is not allowed expression; Henri decides to think of it as just a holiday because he does not want to distress Marguerite. So when she has gone and the separation is irrevocable, Henri is faced with the grief. His experience of her absence is like the grief of a death: he calls and imagines she replies, he expects her to be in the next room and realizes she is not. He says that part of him has gone, but there has been no goodbye. On the other hand, it is not the grief of bereavement, because he has the distress of speaking to her across an ocean, and knowing her unhappiness. She is physically absent, but psychologically present. He is very sad, and there is no one to acknowledge or validate this complicated grief. Such ambiguous loss and grief is a heavy load to carry alone. There is no social network and no family system to support him in the tasks of meaning-making and grieving.

Isolation and existential loneliness

Henri loves to talk. He refers to this often, but this is an isolating and lonely journey. During the year Marguerite has been taken out nearly every day, shopping, to church and church meetings, or for coffee with her friend. Henri does not drive far, is taken for necessary shopping and appointments by a Community Service employee, and occasionally by his son for a meal. Early in the year he meets a friend weekly or fortnightly when he can, and this is his only real opportunity to talk. He is distressed when Marguerite is upset and refuses to talk to him; he still enjoys conversation with her, even if he sees it as meaningless chatter. He misses her when she is out. When she relocates to Canada, his loneliness is palpable. In the isolation of his small home, he faces the loss of his identity as husband, companion, caregiver, and independent home owner; and alone he faces the task of reconstructing his life and identity in what he pictures as an alien and prison-like context.

Therapeutic talking

Not only does Henri love to relate socially, but also talking is the outlet for his emotions. He says he is unable to talk to his family. When he tries to tell his son how it is for him, his son says he has no answers and "turns the page." In relating this and its impact, his body language conveys his pent-up emotions, as he holds his breath. In fact, he analogizes talking as breathing; for him, talking releases the tension within that needs to come out. However, his circumstances largely deprive him of this outlet. He values the empathy offered by his friend whose wife has dementia, and he appreciates the opportunities to talk about the journey with the researcher. Then, he says, he can breathe.

A spiritual journey

Meaning-making is recognized as a spiritual task. Henri cannot make sense of his experience. Initially, he is grateful that he has had a good life for eighty-three years, and cheerfully says he accepts what comes, the ups and the downs. He concludes his first interview on a very positive note, indicating that his purpose, in which God sustains him, is to care for Marguerite. Six months later, he suggests that God keeps him going—and he is a fighter. By the end of the year's journey, his purpose has been lost. He sees nothing to keep him going, and no reason to live. He has no incentive or encouragement to find purpose or meaning in the journey ahead, and he suggests that a person should have the choice to end his life. He still prays, as he has done throughout the year, especially for Marguerite. To some extent, his spiritual life has been sustained in the last few months of the year by a friend, a Christian pastor who has visited to share Holy Communion with them both, but Henri has had no opportunity to talk with him about his struggles. He has no connection with a church community. He stopped attending public worship some time earlier because of the frustration of being unable to hear what was said. Nobody from his church visited him.

Spiritual distress results from a loss of meaning, a loss of connectedness with others, and an inner disharmony and disconnectedness. Whether Henri is able to move beyond his spiritual distress to find meaning in his journey and purpose to take him forward will most likely depend on whether someone gives him permission and opportunity to talk, to "breathe out" what is bottled up within him, to find meaning in the confusion, and to connect with his grief, his despair, his God, and himself.

Elaine's Story

Profile

Elaine, a retired nurse, and Colin, formerly an accountant in a senior managerial position, have been married fifty-five years. The first interview with Elaine occurs about six months after Colin's diagnosis of Alzheimer's Disease, a diagnosis that greatly surprised their long-time family doctor, who had interpreted Colin's symptoms as depression during Elaine's treatment for a serious illness two years earlier. Elaine now makes all the decisions, helps Colin with his self-care, and performs the household tasks. The daily challenges are stressful. Colin is distressed about the jobs he is no longer able to complete; and the losses and fluctuations in his functioning are difficult for Elaine.

Elaine maintains other interests, coordinating a church ladies group and a community group for lonely elderly (though, she reflects, her current minister does not see much value in that). She also has a good network of friends, and enjoys her role as mother and grandmother. At the same time, she makes the most of what she and Colin still have, and engages in caregiving to the best of her ability. She says that anti-depressants are helping her. She values quiet times, prays often for patience and understanding, and maintains connection with the church to which she and Colin have belonged for some years. Colin no longer attends church regularly. There have been a couple of helpful pastoral visits where Colin has been included.

About six months later, Colin's memory has deteriorated further, and this has brought greater challenges. Elaine has to help more with his basic daily self-care, and the unsettling fluctuations in his functioning continue. Communication has become more difficult. Elaine's hearing is not good, Colin's voice has become very soft, he cannot explain what he wants, Elaine cannot always guess, and they both become frustrated. She still tries to cope, with patience and a positive approach, but sometimes she gets upset and angry. She acknowledges how different from her past nursing this experience is, of caring "24/7" for her husband, the home, and herself.

Outside connections are becoming more tenuous. She maintains her involvement in the groups she coordinates, but thinks she may have to relinquish one of these. Apart from one friend on a similar journey, friends offer very little understanding or support and there is withdrawal, for which Elaine blames herself. Since the relocation of the former pastoral care coordinator in her church, there have been no further pastoral visits. At times there are encouraging emails from one person in her church.

Another six months later, the situation has changed significantly. Elaine has had serious illness, a week in hospital, and several weeks' convalescence. She received two pastoral visits in hospital, which really encouraged her. Colin has been in residential respite care during her illness, and now comes home for some days each week. Practical government-funded support is being provided, her family has been practically supportive, and Elaine's friends have rallied around.

Interpretive Analysis

Loss and holding on

Elaine's sense of loss deepens throughout the year, but in the journey so far, she tries to hold on to who her husband has been and to their present life together. She misses his companionship, and sharing with him the joy of the family's achievements and milestones such as their fifty-fifth wedding anniversary. She finds it difficult to accept the contrast between the competent and clever person she has known, and Colin as he is now. In these losses, she identifies hurt and disappointment. The losses increase, and six months later, it is her husband himself whom she feels she has lost. At the end of the year, she reflects again that she has lost her husband and this is a grieving process. Across the year, her initial unwillingness to think about potential losses gives way to accepting an anticipated move for Colin into permanent care, and, looking further forward, to imagining his death as putting away his body, possibly with some sense of relief. However, at the same time she clings to their relationship with firm commitment. Elaine also holds on to connections and roles in her family, church, and community. In the losses so far, she holds on to her own identity and purpose.

Ambiguity and ambivalence

The experience of simultaneous losing and holding on gives rise to a striking element in Elaine's narrative: the seesaw of the affective and the cognitive. Particularly in the first interview, while acknowledging the distress of the journey, she counters every negative with a positive statement. She struggles with what has happened and looks for reasons; but she conveys a positive attitude and verbalizes acceptance. She challenges the unfairness of dementia after they have done "all the right things," but is quick to say that she does not blame God. She draws strength from her faith, but she is not afraid to tell God that at times the journey is almost too much. She acknowledges the loss of her husband as he has been, but alternately clings tightly to what they still have and to making the most of the good days, the good times, the shared events, the surprising flashes of memory. She finds the ambiguity of the daily fluctuations and these flashes of the past bewildering and frustrating, but she repeatedly says she "goes with the flow."

Ambiguity in the losses and ambivalence of affect are recognized as characteristic of the dementia journey; and being able to hold both sides of the experience concurrently and live with the ambiguity without trying to resolve it is the key to resilience and coping.[18] Elaine verbalizes her ambivalent feelings and is ready to tell her story as it is for her, without trying to suppress either side or reconcile the ambiguously opposing sides of loss

18. Boss, *Loss, Trauma*, 16–17.

and holding on. Her determined coping with the increasing demands and grief is the outcome.

Coping

Elaine's coping is achieved through her persistent use of cognitive, affective, and spiritual strategies. She employs positive self-talk, and counterbalances this with the expression of her emotions privately and with one friend who understands. She searches to name these emotions honestly. She is able to laugh as she narrates incidents that could be very frustrating, and to acknowledge the times when she becomes intensely frustrated. She says that she cries, and sometimes sulks, and talks out her frustration and sadness with her friend. Her spiritual life sustains her in the day-to-day challenges; hers is an intrinsic faith, and she prays in the midst of the turmoil. She uses Scriptures to reassure her, but is honest with God when the reality seems to contradict her beliefs. She values quiet times and prayer, and she can still attend public worship. There is a sense of inner harmony as she copes with the vicissitudes of the journey. Nonetheless, that coping is stretched beyond Elaine's physical capacity, and she suffers serious illness.

Purpose and meaning

Elaine acknowledges that she has no answers as to why they are facing this journey. She initially looks for some possible connection with Colin's not liking his profession and with his retrenchment, but she cannot make sense of it all. Amid the absence of answers, however, she has a clear sense of purpose and meaning in the journey. She is committed to Colin and to their marriage, and articulates her purpose: caring for Colin at home as long as possible, making his life as comfortable as possible, and making the most of what they still have. Her goal is to do the best that she can do. At this stage she continues to balance other purposes beyond her caring, seeking to fulfill her role in the family and enhance the lives of people in the community and the church.

Caregiving: A Lived Experience

Network changes

The year's journey is informative concerning Elaine's network support. Initially she is reluctant to access the practical support she knows is available, because she sees that as an acknowledgment of the next stage of Colin's decline. At the first interview, she feels a sense of belonging in her Christian community and a network of good friends, and she had felt supported by a few pastoral visits that included Colin, until they ceased. Their friends' early support disappears as Colin's condition deteriorates and the friends fail to understand the challenges. Some do not respond to her phone calls and messages and are busy with their own lives, and there is disconnection and withdrawal. The lack of understanding is starkly indicated by such comments as one friend's question (after over two years of the journey) as to when Colin will get better. At this stage, Elaine feels a significant absence of support or empathy. Her involvement with the ladies group gives her connection with the flow of other people's lives as she listens, and after her own illness, it gives her opportunities to talk. After this physical illness, she is emotionally buoyed by the care of friends and family and the pastoral hospital visits.

Talking and support

Across the year, there is little opportunity for Elaine to verbalize her questions or articulate her grief. There is no mention of empathic listening, apart from reference to sharing with a friend in a similar situation. While initially she believes that the most effective support would be someone to talk to, six months later she expresses doubt about this. It is the lack of empathy in her friendship network that now causes Elaine uncertainty about what would help emotionally or spiritually: "they don't understand." The pastoral and friendship support she receives in her own serious illness makes a significant difference to her well-being; it moves her (at least while she is ill) from a place of isolation and withdrawal to a place of feeling connected and valued. Though Elaine does not draw comparisons, this experience of support suggests contrasting responses to the dementia journey and physical illness, the difference of absence and presence, ignorance and understanding, neglect and care. Empathic failure in her church friendship network attends the dementia journey.

Sustaining Persons, Grieving Losses

Lorraine's Story

Profile

Lorraine is pragmatic, unemotional, and determined. While working full-time, she has been caring for her seventy-two year old mother, Dorothy, for six years, since an accident produced or revealed early stage dementia. There have been huge practical challenges since Lorraine facilitated a move for her mother to live near her. Lorraine has a sister, her mother's "favorite daughter," who has not seen her mother for three years, and the whole load falls on Lorraine's shoulders, though she has her own adult family, grandchildren, and full-time work.

During the journey Dorothy has had major health issues and significant lengths of time in hospital, with a heart condition, dementia, and recently diagnosed epilepsy. Lorraine has been engaged in ongoing battles with hospitals, doctors, and social workers, who insist that Dorothy cannot look after herself, that Lorraine is not looking after her properly, and that Dorothy should go into a nursing home. Lorraine has been extremely frustrated about not being listened to at the hospitals concerning her mother's usual level of competence and independence. She has been unable to get information from the hospitals about available community support, instead being handed a folder about aged care centers. She has finally found the internet and her neighbor to be better sources of information. There has been increased time pressure because of the hospital's insistence that before her mother is discharged, Lorraine must provide documentary evidence that Dorothy will be in Day Respite five days a week. It has been "a logistic nightmare" for Lorraine to fit in making these arrangements, visits to hospital, and her work; but she is determined that Dorothy will not go into permanent care until Lorraine knows that this is necessary. Her goal is that her mother will have dignity and quality of life as long as possible.

By taking Dorothy for a consultation with Lorraine's own family doctor, the medication dosages were found to be incorrect, and with that addressed, Dorothy has gained mobility and some independence. She now attends respite centers daily—except occasionally when she absconds and catches a bus to a large retail center where she has formerly built a network of shop-employee friends in her years addicted to shopping. Lorraine employs an early morning care-giver for Dorothy until the respite center bus arrives, and cares for her after work till her mother's bedtime. She is re-teaching her mother to sew, as her considerable skill in that area has been forgotten.

The stress is ongoing, but Lorraine copes. In the past, her wood lathe has been her outlet—she "massacres wood"—but the time pressures and Dorothy's presence have made her hobby impossible. She says she and her mother have always been alienated, but she assumes that the occasional violence toward her is because Dorothy does not recognize her. She accepts with humor the occasional lack of recognition. Lorraine says her adult children are supportive, and she enjoys her work. She has never had involvement in a church, but she has her own spiritual beliefs and quiet times that give her strength.

Eight months later, there have been changes. While Lorraine acknowledges her mother's ongoing cognitive deterioration, there have been health and mobility improvements. Dorothy is able to dress herself and make a cup of tea, and the doctor is surprised. Lorraine tells him, "we pushed the exercise; we pushed the sewing to use her hands; we pushed the mind with word puzzles." In all, there have been seven hospital stays, but none in the past four months, and there is now cooperation and support from the assigned hospital doctor. There is also increased support from the Community Care provider. Another change is planned: Lorraine is about to buy a larger home, so that her mother can be under the same roof but still have some independence. There are still challenges. Her mother becomes abusive when Lorraine sets limits on her obsessive spending. Lorraine is still not free to pursue her woodturning, because of her care commitments. She herself has been unwell for three weeks, but otherwise all is manageable.

Four months further on, Dorothy's cognition has deteriorated, but her health has remained stable. She is still sewing, though Lorraine has to prompt her diplomatically or she forgets. The move to a new home has not yet eventuated. Because the employed morning care-giver has been away, Lorraine has been getting up at 3 a.m. for the last three weeks in order to fit her work in around her mother's care. There have been no new challenges, and Dorothy, while at times still abusive, is quieter and more tractable. As Lorraine reflects on her years of caring, she repeats that her life has been on hold, in fact, she has not had a life during that time. She has not been able to go on holidays or outings as she previously did. She takes satisfaction in her mother's continuing independence and level of functioning, though there is no gratitude from Dorothy. Lorraine's family values, learnt from her grandparents, still give meaning to her caregiving role.

Sustaining Persons, Grieving Losses

Interpretive Analysis

Purpose

Lorraine's clear sense of purpose drives and sustains her through a very challenging journey. There are three tightly bound strands of purpose: doing what she believes is best for her mother, making the most of what she has, and being family. It is her firm belief that independence and dignity are best maintained outside nursing homes, and she battles for her mother's independence. Her unswerving determination about this has a high cost to Lorraine in terms of her time, finances, and well-being. However, she will not be diverted from this goal and has put her own life "on hold" for her mother's sake. The value she places on family bonds drives her to model commitment and sacrifice for her own family, although she did not have such modeling in her childhood. This she sees as the right way, and she will not do less. Her loss of a grandchild in the previous year has heightened her awareness that life is precarious, and has reinforced her commitment to making the most of family relationships while there is time. This gives meaning to her journey.

Unconditional love

Lorraine's caregiving provides a salutary example of unconditional love. She repeatedly refers, and apparently without bitterness, to the long-term alienation and conflict in her relationship with her mother, and she has no expectations of positive change in this. And yet, in her narration of their interactions she reveals affection, humor, and acceptance. She positively attributes Dorothy's violence and aggression to her failure to recognize Lorraine, and she copes with Dorothy's sarcasm and nastiness, as she has always done, by switching off. She accepts good-naturedly Dorothy's criticism and lack of appreciation of her efforts, and in the bantering there appears to be good humor rather than malice. There is no evidence in Lorraine's narrative of expectations of any reward for her personal and financial sacrifice, except the satisfaction of knowing that she has done the best she can, has achieved the highest quality of life for her mother's last years, and has made the most of the time.

Caregiving: A Lived Experience

Positive Appraisals

It is interesting that—while there are numerous references to relational conflict with her mother since her early childhood, and several comments about her mother's favoritism toward Lorraine's absent and unsupportive sister—Lorraine interprets her mother's actions and responses toward her positively. Dorothy's abuse does not devastate her, as she does not perceive this as an attack on her own identity. When Dorothy thinks that Lorraine is someone else's kind daughter and that Lorraine is neglecting her, Lorraine accepts this with good humor. Resentment is apparently not a factor in her caregiving, and any frustration is directed toward external obstacles in the way of maintaining her mother's quality of life.

Personal Identity

Lorraine has a clearly defined sense of self, secure in who she is. This is evident in her acceptance of her mother's failure at times to recognize her or appreciate what she is sacrificing for Dorothy's well-being. The social workers' assessment of Lorraine's caregiving as inadequate for Dorothy's needs might have undermined her confidence, but it has not; rather, it makes her more determined to fight for Dorothy's rights. This self-confidence enables her to achieve her goal of increased independence for her mother through medication changes and hard work on Lorraine's part. Identity is recognized as being socially formed and nourished, and Lorraine is not dependent on the relationship with her mother for the nourishment of her identity; she has other family roles as mother and grandmother, and work relationships where she is valued. It might be inferred from her story that Lorraine's identity has developed in spite of, rather than because of, her relationship as daughter.

Support

Lorraine has had limited support in the journey. She was initially frustrated because she could not find what practical support was available or how to access any. She has given no thought to what emotional support is available or might be helpful. Although she is very used to being independent and coping, at the first interview she has been under severe pressure. In this interview she speaks for an hour almost without taking breath, and her body language suggests increasing trust and relaxation throughout the hour. She sees herself as a good listener, and listens to her neighbor, employer, and workmates; but she is able to switch off to their emotions. In the last interview, she reflects that she is using what she has learnt on this journey to support others in their stressful situations. She has always coped, and does not look to others for support. In interviews a year apart, she refers to "unloading" to her dog.

Coping

Lorraine's coping strategies in the face of high emotional and physical demands are interesting. She deals cognitively with the challenges, and sets aside or redirects her emotions. A deep mark has been left on her by the sudden deaths of both her husband and her father, where there was no opportunity for Lorraine to say goodbye. Her rather understated description of this as "disheartening" is indicative of her ways of handling emotions. In general, she deals pragmatically with potentially traumatic situations by minimizing or switching off to her emotions, relegating them to the background to be dealt with in her own way, at a later time. For her, woodturning is an important outlet for frustration. However, this outlet has been unavailable to her before and throughout this stressful year. The force of the underlying emotions is directed toward positive action for her mother, whom she dreads losing unexpectedly, having found her on the floor in a coma more than once. She uses her energy to fight professionals who misinterpret the situation, to resist the deterioration in her mother's condition, and to make the most of the time. Wry humor provides relief in what might be very stressful interactions with her mother. She sees work and its problems as a diversion from caregiving stresses. It appears that an early life of fighting adversity has given her invaluable resilience in this journey.

Spirituality

Lorraine's spirituality sustains her. She finds meaning in family values, and in doing the very best she can. The caring takes its toll, but she employs spiritual strategies, seeing quiet times for unloading as vital, and believing in "something" from which she draws strength to keep going. She reflects on the importance of this aspect of coping, suggesting that she would otherwise "probably collapse."

Caregiving: A Lived Experience

Beverley's Story

Profile

Beverley and Tom have been married forty-five years. Tom's dementia was diagnosed by a geriatrician two years ago, when Beverley pushed for a referral following a frustrating year in which their family doctor had brushed aside her concerns about Tom's memory as "just aging." At this stage Beverley adopts the same attitude toward Tom's condition as has brought her through two bouts of life-threatening illness: "Well, this is it. I've just got to get through it."

Life is not as they had expected. Before his retirement from his profession, Tom had looked forward to being involved with the "Men's Shed" with a group of men at their church, and to having Beverley around all the time. They had both looked forward to touring around Australia. An active sixty-six-year-old, she had pictured herself continuing in her various roles in the church and community—among others she has been secretary of a school "Parents and Citizens Association" for over thirty years, is a committee member of a service club, and belongs to a local theater group. She previously managed the church office for some years, and was involved in the Parish Council.

The dementia journey thus far has been quite challenging for Beverley. Having to carry the whole load of work, planning, and decision-making has been compounded by the constancy of Tom's forgetting, questioning, and repetition, and these have brought her to a state of extreme frustration. She is frustrated by Tom's lack of initiative, his withdrawal from outside life, and his dependence on her. She resents his clinging to her, and feels that her life has to be lived around caring for him. She has relinquished some of her outside activities, but firmly intends to maintain her lifestyle, interests, and outlets.

Beverley has not accessed support. Shortly after the diagnosis, her family doctor attempted to contact an Alzheimer's support organization about a brief respite for her, with no response, and so she is not interested in an Alzheimer's support group. There has been a vague suggestion that several caregivers with partners with dementia in their congregation might form a support group. She does not feel supported by her church community, in which they have both actively participated for over thirty years. She does have a friend, also caring for a husband with dementia, with whom she is able to share her frustrations. She mentions that her family is supportive, though only one daughter and her family live close by.

Six months later, Tom's memory has deteriorated further, and he has become more dependent. His confusion has increased, and he constantly questions Beverley about upcoming activities, family relationships, and familiar tasks like making a cup of tea. It is an effort to persuade him to go out, so she pushes him only if she is sure he will enjoy the outing. However, she cannot converse with him about it afterwards, because it is forgotten. Beverley is beginning to accept that he *cannot* rather that *will not* remember, but she still struggles to realize his limitations. Rather than the earlier approach of "something comes, something goes," she acknowledges that this is a difficult journey that will not become easier. Beverley now has some depression, which she fights. She misses normal conversation and companionship with Tom. She is reluctant to look ahead or access help, as she sees doing so as acknowledging the next stage. She prefers to deal only with the present, clinging to activities and commitments that give meaning to her life.

Support continues to be minimal. Apart from the daughter who lives near, and her friend in a similar caring role, there is no one else. Nobody at church seems interested. The men of the church men's group say they should visit Tom, but they do not. She sees the absence of corporate prayer for specific needs in the congregation as symptomatic of a general lack of support. Whereas she has previously attended the church service weekly without fail, she now finds excuses.

Another six months later, Beverley is still struggling to accept the reality of Tom's condition, to remember that he *cannot* remember, and to accept his limitations. There has been further cognitive deterioration, and there is now little recognition of anyone beyond the immediate family. Beverley has faced grief alone. Their much loved old pet cat has died on Tom's lap, an event he didn't remember even immediately afterwards. This is distressing, as it underlines the loss of companionship and shared memories. Her depression has increased and the doctor has offered her antidepressants, but she is coping without.

She is now able to verbalize some positive aspects of her journey. Tom's is only a memory and comprehension problem and he is still able to enjoy outings with her, even if he forgets immediately. She is finding life manageable at present.

Caregiving: A Lived Experience

Interpretive Analysis

Cognitive appraisals, emotional responses

Beverley's experience of the journey so far has not been comfortable. Her appraisal of Tom's behaviors contributes to some resentment. She sees Tom's clinging as an extension of his earlier tendency to want her to himself and to discourage the social interactions that she had initiated for them as a couple. She views his need to be "pushed" as an amplified form of the lack of initiative that became apparent, she believes, after a traumatic event at work some years ago. This history adds to her frustration. The appraisal of Tom's lack of understanding and initiative as an *unwillingness* to cooperate increases Beverley's frustration, and she seeks to control his functioning and memory, to insist he give her space, and to "make" him remember and understand and stop asking questions. The failure of these strategies leads to a sense of powerlessness and frustration. During the year, there is a gradual shift in Beverley's appraisals. Twelve months later, she acknowledges the uncontrollability of the situation, and recognizes that it is she who has to make the cognitive adjustments, though there is still some ambiguity about what Tom *will* not or *cannot* do. As her appraisals change and the degree of acceptance increases, the emotion that Beverley sees as frustration and Tom hears as anger is lessened. She has moved gradually to an acceptance of Tom's increasing limitations.

Ambiguity and ambivalence

As the year progresses and denial is replaced by greater acceptance, Beverley becomes more aware of Tom's increasing losses, including his loss of memory, the loss of talents like his music, and the loss of any memory of faith or church connection. She struggles with the ambiguity of the loss, as he still looks like the person she has known for over fifty years. The losses in their relationship, particularly in companionship and shared memories, leave her feeling very isolated. There is ambivalence in this experience, however; she feels alone in an "isolation bubble" and yet simultaneously trapped by his clinging like a vine. The loss and ambivalence are poignantly highlighted with the death of their cat. She has anticipated with dread her husband's possibly repeated expressions of grief, but when he immediately forgets the loss she is both relieved and disappointed, and she is left "in limbo" with her own unshared and unacknowledged grief.

Sustaining Persons, Grieving Losses

The ambiguity of many losses and the ambivalence of the feelings are a difficult experience for someone who sees herself as very practical, who likes everything clear-cut and straightforward. She experiences anticipatory grief, reluctantly recognizing that she will have to sell their home and downsize to reduce her workload, and she is concerned about how Tom will feel about going into a residential aged care center when the time comes. She is aware of how different the future will be from their planned future, but she would rather deal pragmatically with the present, frustrating as it is, than think about the future losses. Beverley views herself as unemotional and strong, coping rather than crying. In the gradual and potential loss of social connection and community purposes, there is still an unwillingness to reflect on the losses and uncertainties. Beverley says that, while talking about them may be helpful, it is disturbing to think about things that she would prefer not to face. A close relationship has been found in dementia caregiving between depressive symptoms and grief,[19] and it is noteworthy that the increasing awareness of ambiguous, ongoing loss coincides with Beverley's increasing depression. When and how the grief of the ambiguous but significant losses will be processed is an open question.

Goals and purpose

With the shift toward acceptance across the year, there is a gradual shift in Beverley's goals. From clinging to her own lifestyle as the solution to the situation, six months later she moves to just trying to cope. Another six months on, Beverley has moved on from looking for answers, wondering what caused the dementia, and wishing for a cure, to the position of making cognitive changes to accept the situation and make the best of it, appreciating that there are many others coping with much greater challenges than just their partner's loss of memory. She does not, however, verbalize any sense of purpose in caregiving. Thus far her strong sense of purpose has been found in serving her community and church.

Identity and connection

In the caring journey, Beverley's identity is important to her. She feels as though a clinging vine is wrapping itself around her, gradually taking over

---

19. Sanders and Adams, "Grief and Depression," 293–94.

her life and threatening to cut her off from her past activities, her present lifestyle, and her planned future. While struggling against this, she at the same time feels she has lost her companion and gained a role as "just a carer." She holds tightly to her life as it has been, to her outside roles and interests and her own space; but the more she seeks to keep her identity and her space intact, the more she feels impinged upon. Her social connections and her church and community service have contributed significantly to her sense of who she is, and she indicates that she needs these connections to sustain her, even if her husband insists on withdrawing. On the other hand, as the year unfolds, she experiences a growing sense of disconnection from the church that has been so significant to her identity.

Support

Following a change in church staff, Beverley perceives the level of support for herself and Tom from their faith community of many years to be minimal. People occasionally enquire after Tom but have never visited him, though he was actively involved and serving in the church until the onset of dementia. She feels there has been a shift in attitudes to pastoral care in her church in recent years, from a time when "they really cared about their people." She feels some rejection on behalf of Tom and herself, but she does not expect that people should "put themselves out" to support her. Beverley expresses the wish, in two visits, for tangible support through occasional meals. She regrets the absence of prayer in church services for congregational members in need, and latterly feels that her absence from participation might go unnoticed, though she has had, and still has, significant roles. She wonders where God is in it, but indicates that her faith is all she has to hold on to; and she is quick to establish that she does not blame God for her circumstances. While Beverley says that she thinks her own faith and prayers help her in the journey, her practice of faith appears to be more focused on participation in public worship and involvement in the church community. This now requires effort on her part, and there is a change from her patterns of regular attendance to wondering about withdrawing altogether. Research suggests that for caregivers of persons with dementia, both intrinsic and extrinsic elements of faith appear to be related to how they respond emotionally, with higher levels of support from their religious community being associated with lower levels of anger.[20] With the sense

20. Marquez-Gonzalez et al., "Anger, Spiritual Meaning," 183–85.

of being unsupported and possibly invisible, and with the effort required to maintain connection, it is unsurprising that Beverley's anger and then depression have not been ameliorated.

Beverley expresses uncertainty about what emotional and spiritual support might be helpful. The suggested Alzheimer's support group has held no attraction because of her feeling "let down." Beverley wonders whether the vaguely proposed church support group might have helped. While she finds it helpful to talk with her friend facing similar challenges, that connection has diminished because of caregiving demands. She is ambivalent about the value of talking because she feels that people other than caregivers do not understand—and anyway, she prefers to be practical rather than reflective. In light of this, however, it is interesting to observe her readiness to speak of her journey three times for an hour at a time, and to note the therapeutic effect of this. Particularly in the first interview, there is a dramatic shift from initially expressing intense frustration with Tom, to acknowledging how it might be for him, and then to reflecting on how her responses to him might change. It is worth considering whether regular empathic listening might have diffused the ongoing frustration and enabled Beverley much earlier to explore her grief, move from denial toward acceptance, and discover purpose in the caregiving role that has been thrust on her. It is also worth reflecting on how this might have affected Tom's well-being.

Mary's Story

Profile

Mary, a gentle, quietly spoken woman in her early eighties, has been married for over fifty-five years to James. Over twenty years ago, James had his first stroke with associated cognitive impairment. This condition, together with their son's intellectual impairment, has placed her in a long-term caregiving role. In recent years the son has moved from home to supported accommodation with five hours per day of employed caregiver support, and Mary is on call for him at all other times. Mary herself has had a stroke that has affected her vision, and she suffers from arthritis. Four years ago, one of their daughters died in an accident. Another daughter was diagnosed with cancer during that same year, and the cancer has recently recurred. A son lives quite close; others are further away and without transport. James's memory deterioration has escalated over the past two years.

At the first interview, Mary faces many conflicting demands, and she is exhausted. In her daughter's fight against cancer, the practical and emotional support of attending weekly medical appointments and chemotherapy sessions falls on Mary's shoulders. At present this weekly day-long visit occupies her "respite" day, when her husband attends a day respite center run by a community care organization. Mary no longer has her former monthly social connections with a group of friends because of James's condition and her friends' discomfort in his presence, and she is unable to go out alone because of her vision problems. Her only regular "social" contact is with employees from the community care organization, who make brief daily visits to provide healthcare. Her isolation has produced a longing to be involved in the normal flow of life beyond the limits of home, hospital, and shopping center.

James's life is less confined. He has been able to maintain some of his earlier connections and roles, because of the support of men in a service club he belongs to and the Returned Servicemen's League. With transport provided by other members, he attends weekly meetings and receives affirmation and acceptance there. As well as a day per week at the respite center, James is taken on an enjoyable four-hour weekly outing to give Mary "respite" at home. Mary longs for such outings. He also enjoys "pottering" in the garden, and watching his many favorite television programs.

The future is uncertain. Against the background of the earlier loss of their first daughter, where grief almost overwhelmed Mary, there is the very present fear of "what's around the corner" for her daughter with cancer. There is uncertainty too about the future with her husband. Because of his insistence that she promise not to put him into a residential aged care center, even for residential respite care, for her there is a sense of being trapped in her situation for an unknown duration.

Mary seeks to cope by accepting what cannot be changed and working on what can be changed. She is ambivalent about seeking support. She has always perceived this as weakness and an indication of not coping, but on the other hand, she thinks that maybe she should seek some support from her church or the chaplain of the community care organization. She says that her faith and religious practices enable her to cope. She prays the "Serenity Prayer" daily, says the Rosary every night, and finds strength in going to Mass when her son takes her.

Six months later, there is both change and continuity in the journey. The family demands are ongoing, her daughter's health issues are still physically and emotionally challenging for Mary, and the fourth anniversary of her other daughter's death confronts her with painful memories of her loss. Busyness and exhaustion have increased and Mary's own health has deteriorated, with decreased mobility and further deterioration of her vision, and a consequent loss of self-confidence. There has been further deterioration in her husband's cognition and his managing of daily self-care. He needs more help and supervision, which he strongly resists. Apparently oblivious of the chaos and stress surrounding his personal world, he has increasing expectations that everything must be exactly as he wants it. Consequently, anger has added to the stress.

Over the six months, there has been change in the support received. Interestingly, none of the significant gain in support has been at Mary's instigation. Family support and outings have increased, and there is monthly connection with the respite center at a morning tea for clients with dementia and their caregivers. Mary really enjoys this. There is now meaningful connection with a former friend facing similar challenges in caring for her husband who also has early-stage dementia. This friend takes Mary out weekly for coffee, and this makes a very real difference to Mary's quality of life.

At the same time, there has been a loss of spiritual support. Connection with the church has disappeared because her son no longer attends Mass, and Mary cannot attend alone. There is a longing for Holy Communion, and for a conversation with the priest. Mary doubts whether support would be provided, in light of her several months' absence. She still has faith and prays, but rather than strength coming from religious contacts, it is now the social contact that enables her to face the week.

About seven months later, there have been major changes in the journey. Their daughter has died, and now the daughter's son (with a disability) lives with them in their small home, with his own need for fixed routines. Mary has not allowed herself to grieve, as she has to keep going. She has been unable to share her grief with her husband, who does not connect with the loss—an absence of emotional response that Mary attributes to his dementia. Instead of shared grieving, Mary faces her husband's expectation that everything continue as it was before, with him as the focus.

There have been other changes too. The outings have ceased, because her son is now very busy with a new partner, and her friend is no longer available because of care demands. With her vision problems, Mary is too frightened to go out alone or even to walk across the street to a friendly neighbor. The monthly outing to the respite center morning tea continues. Apart from this and taking a taxi to necessary appointments, Mary stays home.

In her losses, Mary has at last sought help. Since their second daughter's death, she has gone to her church to ask about possible occasional transport to Mass and to speak to the priest, but this has been "disappointing." He offered only platitudes. In her grief, Mary has also tried to talk to her doctor, but left very angry because of his lack of interest in her needs. She shares with the researcher her past (and now lost) dreams of building a counseling business, and her longing that her long-ago achievement of a counseling diploma might be recognized, at least at her funeral.

Interpretive Analysis

Personal identity

Mary feels that her very "self" has been lost. Her hopes for her own life, her gifts, and her preferences have been set aside, and her circumstances have deprived her of opportunities for rebuilding her identity and her personal world. In this caregiving journey, she has faced major changes: significant losses in the family structure, the loss of her friendship network and her creative crafts, and latterly, the connection with her church. James's advancing dementia has brought a gradual and ambiguous loss of her husband as he was, with occasional bewildering flashes of his past self that bring surprise and pride. While she holds on to elements of her personal identity, such as her family values, her faith, and her Irish heritage, she fears that she is losing other elements of herself, such as her memory and her ability to express herself—she used to do public speaking, she says, and now she cannot even find the word she wants in conversation. There is hidden sadness that her skills and gifts have not been used and that her hopes for herself cannot be realized.

Personal identity is socially formed, in the marriage relationship and with family, friends, and the wider social context, and we need a social context in which we can interpret change in order to assimilate it.[21] For Mary, all these contexts have been eroded or lost. She still misses the daughter

---

21. Marris, "Holding onto Meaning," 15–16.

with whom, until five years ago, she could share her feelings; and her earlier friends have gone. In the years before this and through this year, there has been nobody offering an opportunity for Mary to express and explore her feelings, to narrate and see the reality of her experience, and to reflect on her application of her long-held philosophy and beliefs, apart from a friend in a similar caring role in a brief interlude of empathic connection, and an unknown researcher. There has been no context for her to rebuild her identity.

A CONFINED WORLD

After many years on her caregiving journey, Mary feels trapped. Her life has been shaped by her context and the demands of caring for her husband with dementia, her son with a disability, and her daughter with terminal illness. Companionship and emotional connection have largely disappeared. Holding values where the family is paramount, Mary's own world has been consumed by her husband's world, where he is central and wields control. Her most recent challenge is to accommodate another rigidly defined world of routine, in which their grandson lives. For Mary, there is no escape beyond the walls of her home, which she feels are closing in on her; and her only ongoing connections are phone calls with a daughter and the brief daily conversations with employed caregivers. She eagerly looks forward to their visits, but feels guilty about this because they have told her that friendship with clients is frowned upon by their organization.

GRIEF AND LONELINESS

There is no context where Mary might express and receive validation of her grief, or process the challenges that her losses bring to her assumptive world, or make meaning in her journey. Such a context is unavailable in family, church, and with the family doctor. And for Mary there is no other world, except the shower and the ironing room where she sometimes allows herself the private "luxury" of tears. Caregivers experience disenfranchised grief, in the absence of social and family validation,[22] but Mary's circumstances have extended the range of her disenfranchised grief beyond her husband's losses, to include her other losses of family, connections, hopes,

---

22. Doka, "Disenfranchised Grief," 224.

and self. Her experience in these losses is manifest as a heart-wrenching existential loneliness, and a deep longing for connection, meaningful human contact, and acknowledgment of her losses and her identity.

Coping

Mary takes the Serenity Prayer as her foundation for coping. She has prayed the prayer daily for many years, and seeks to live by it; but as she shares her story and opens up her world to someone who listens, she hears her own story and sees inconsistencies in her application of the prayer. She decides that she has been worrying and living on the side of what she cannot change, and that there is another side, where she does not have to accept without question, and where she might have the courage to make changes. However, the occasional and surprising reappearances of her husband's former self and the ambiguity of his level of competence—with the uncertainty about what *he* can control—blur the line between what she needs to accept and what she needs to change. The positive changes in support that have occurred during the year have not been at Mary's instigation, and have been, not through her choosing, short lived. The year with its emotional and spiritual challenges has stretched her coping strategies to the limit, but she continues to pray and cling to her faith.

Help-seeking

Mary sees coping and help-seeking as mutually exclusive, and she is used to coping. The concept of seeking help is alien to her, and—with some ambivalence—she resists seeking it. However, her grief in the loss of her first daughter almost overwhelmed her; and when, along with all the other losses, she faces profound grief in the loss of her second daughter, in deep need she seeks help. She ventures beyond the world of her emotionally detached family to seek connection and support. With her disenfranchised grief and spiritual longings, she goes first to her religious community. She is met with unresponsiveness to her practical need of transport to Mass, and with the priest's religious platitudes that deny her her grief. She accepts with resignation not having her needs addressed, deciding that "it's not their fault." It is easier to ignore the challenge to her assumptive world where the church is always right, and she does not allow herself any expression of disappointment or anger. In one more attempt to address her grief, she experiences her doctor's dismissal of her needs in favor of her husband's, and now she allows herself to feel very angry. Failure has greeted Mary's courageous attempts to change what she can. Her attempts to improve her situation have not been fruitful, and the responses to her help-seeking have added to her pain and aloneness.

Spiritual pain and faith

The loss of support of family and friends, the sense of a loss of self, and a disconnection from life are indicators of spiritual distress. Mary, disconnected from the normal flow of life and meaningful relationships and denied a personal identity, experiences loneliness, loss, and longing that constitute spiritual distress. But in her isolation and grief, she clings to her spiritual anchor; she has not lost her faith. It is her intrinsic faith that provides the construct for meaning and identity. In the enforced absence from participation in a faith community, and without sustenance from the sacraments and rituals important to her, she still holds on to her faith and seeks to live in the serenity of acceptance and courage. Even when her courageous attempts to seek empathy, connection, and acknowledgment of her identity bear no fruit, she claims her identity and place in relation to God, and copes in her knowledge that "He's still there . . . I'm still here and I'm coping, um, I talk to him every night."

Empathic listening

Mary knows the value of empathy and longs for it, and she appreciates the significance of being heard. As she verbalizes the pain and distress of the journey, she acknowledges the importance of bringing her experience into the light in order to discover what is happening, how it is affecting her, and what it all means; and she notes the negative effects of holding it within her. Life review is acknowledged as an important activity in the search for meaning, and Mary, having engaged with herself and the researcher in reviewing her journey of caring, seeks to reclaim something of her identity and the meaning of her life. In the last research interview, she brings her lost hopes and dreams for her life from the depths; and immediately after this visit she searches out the symbols of her lost self, her counseling certificates and diplomas from thirty years earlier, in the hope that they will bring recognition of who she is, if only at her funeral. These symbols and the achievements they symbolize are summarily dismissed by her son, as not worth anything more than "pieces of toilet paper." She is left with her loss and longing, but she has been heard—if only by an unknown researcher—and she is very grateful.

Edward's Story

Profile

Edward and Evelyn had been married for over fifty-five years when Evelyn died with advanced dementia. She had been diagnosed with Alzheimer's disease about seven years earlier, and there had been a slow deterioration requiring Edward's caring for her, initially at home and then in an "independent living unit" in a church-affiliated aged care center. Three years after a further move into a dementia unit in the center, Evelyn died with Edward at her side. Two weeks after her death, Edward—a gracious, genteel, retired missionary/minister—speaks of his present experience and, in retrospect, of the dementia journey that he describes as the "long goodbye."

It has been a journey of increasing isolation and loss. The family has been very supportive, with two sons living fairly close, and there is one widowed friend who understands. Otherwise, though surrounded by people, Edward's journey has been a lonely one. He says that, although he began saying goodbye seven years earlier, he has been too busy to grieve during the journey, and anyway he really only began to experience grief near the end. He seeks to be analytical about it now, to think about it logically. In talking about it he uncovers his emotions, but says he will keep them in check till later.

Six months after his wife's death, his grief has taken shape. The experience is one of painful emptiness, punctuated each Tuesday by the vivid memory of the intimate experience of being with his wife at her death. There are other vivid memories too, of the coldness of the last few weeks of her life, not just of winter cold but also of less-than-caring nursing care she received. He is confronted constantly by a large poster with its statement that "the elderly deserve the best" on the wall of the aged care center where he lives, and he struggles with the irony in the light of his recent experience.

In preparation for this interview, Edward has written some reflections. He reads out that in caring for his wife, his own spiritual life has disintegrated. He speaks of maintaining connection, through attendance at services, with the church where he and Evelyn belonged and served for many years; but he has ongoing challenges of trying to connect with his church's corporate life. His health issues have been numerous and demanding. His impaired hearing renders the corporate activities of worship, prayer, and meditation inaudible, and he is frustrated by the failure of worship leaders to articulate clearly. He reflects that pastoral care for the aged "tends to come lower down the list." In his church context, he has not been listened to.

In the loneliness, there are glimmers of light. Edward reminds himself that he has some interest in family events and that there is some purpose in those relationships, even though he says he doesn't grasp those purposes eagerly. He uses a couple of chants that he finds meaningful, and he recites one:

> Calm, Lord, as you still the storm; still me, Lord, keep me from harm.
> Let all the tumult within me cease, and fold me, Lord, in your peace.
> —anonymous prayer, Celtic tradition

Six months later, on the eve of the first anniversary of his wife's death, the emptiness is still there. Time is still measured in weeks since the day of Evelyn's death, which remains a very vivid memory. Life is a matter of fulfilling the requirements to stay alive, though he sees no purpose in going on. The only glimmer of light is "the future hope," but that "doesn't generate anything that I want to go on with."

Connections with his church and faith are somewhat tenuous. He is still frustrated by the fact that he cannot hear what is said in public worship. One person (who tells him she had been greatly helped by him pastorally in a difficult time) has talked with him "a couple of times," and that was meaningful for him, but it is difficult for them to connect because of her busy schedule of providing social care. Otherwise there has been no pastoral support. His mind wanders if he tries to pray, but the chant is meaningful. He still has the faith to find God, at times somewhat to his surprise, in "coincidental" events. Edward reflects on the dementia journey, touching his chest as he describes this as an internally disturbing experience of "watching her gradually falling apart as a person." He indicates that while he earlier dealt with the loss logically, the emotions have now caught up with him.

Caregiving: A Lived Experience

Interpretive Analysis

Loss and grief

Edward's journey has been one of ongoing loss of what has been most significant to him, through the long journey of loss with his wife. In the seven years of caring, any grief was ignored. He himself was not aware of it until near the end of her life, and while he found comfort in the celebration of her life in the funeral service, much of his loss had preceded this time. In the losses there has been an inevitability that has rendered this controlled and competent man powerless, and an unpredictability that has constantly challenged his logical approach. The physical separation that began with Evelyn's entry into a dementia unit in the aged care center has been very painful. Now he faces widowhood, one of the most stressful of life changes, where there is a loss of identity expressed by Edward in terms of half of him being lost.

Edward's assumptive world has been severely challenged. He has lived all his adult life with the belief that the emotions are controllable and that giving way to them is weakness, and his grief confronts this belief. In reflecting just after Evelyn's death that if one did not have a spiritual background one might be angry, he reveals a further tenet of his assumptive world: anger has no place in his spirituality, and by implication is not permitted in his grief. However, Edward's attempts to cope by dealing cognitively with his loss ultimately fail, and his emotions surface during this year of bereavement. The experiences during this year have moved him beyond the "pat answers" that he thinks are expected of him, into the experiential reality of grief and to the honesty of acknowledging that he does not want to go on living.

Existential loneliness

The outworking of Edward's loss and grief is a deep, existential loneliness. This loneliness began with the physical separation three years before his bereavement, and the strong relational connections with his life partner and companion have been gradually eroded. His wife's death leaves a large hole that a year later remains unfilled. His story paints a picture of a grief-stricken man in an empty space, with an existential hollowness within. Edward is painfully conscious of a difference between people's response to physical illness and their response to what he sees as the "nebulous disturbance" and deterioration of the mind. He notes that people are comfortable talking about heart disease and they offer support and a hug in such situations, but they are embarrassed and awkward in enquiring about his journey, and do not hug or want to hear. To this articulate, reserved, but sensitive man for whom physical contact is significant, such distancing is painful. If he had been heard and hugged and embraced in community, the empty space in which he finds himself might have been peopled, and the existential loneliness might have been eased.

Identity and connection

Personal and social meanings enable a person to say "I am here; I am this."[23] What personal and social meanings enable Edward to rebuild a sense of identity, meaning, and place? When the journey of losing has been a long one, where else but in the community that has been the primary social context can significance, place, and belonging be rebuilt? Churches may be, for older cohorts, the most important source of support other than family, especially as people lose their friendship network.[24] It might be expected that Edward's church community should have a central role in this rebuilding process. This man and his wife, his former ministry partner, have served and participated in their local faith community for many years, and connection with this community has been maintained by Edward during the seven years of Evelyn's cognitive deterioration. His own physical challenges are major, and his hearing impairment interferes with social interactions and with spiritual connection in church services and corporate prayers. He faces his bereavement with a sense of disconnection from the community with which he has faithfully maintained physical connection. His church's communal life offers no affirmation or sustenance of who he is, or encouragement in rebuilding his life in the loss of his partner.

Christian community

At present, Edward's Christian community provides him with no sense of belonging. Rather, there is an experience of heightened isolation in the crowd after weekly church, where everyone else's life is moving on, and

---

23. Eisenhander, *Keeping Faith*, 6.
24. Coleman, "Ageing and Personhood," 65–68.

Caregiving: A Lived Experience

Edward feels he needs to escape to the safety of his empty home. The picture is of a community where ministers are very busy doing ministry and where people occasionally open the door to his world only to slam it shut immediately and move on, unwilling to understand or connect with the pain of his journey. He refers to only one pastoral visit immediately after his wife's death, where he experienced the comfort of being heard, a prayer related to his personal needs, and a hug, which was significant. In the absence of ongoing pastoral care, Edward draws the conclusion that he, because he is a retired minister, is expected to cope. He infers that people expect that he should be stronger because of this latter part of his life journey; but his journey has been an experience of diminution rather than growth. There is a marked contrast between Edward's faithful and unconditional love in his marriage till the separation through death, and the disconnection and absence of care from the community of which he is a part.

Spiritual pain

Edward describes his experience of the dementia journey as "internally disturbing," and the sense of emptiness as painful. His physical care for his wife has, he suggests, been accompanied by a disintegration of his spiritual life, with little energy for consistent spiritual practices apart from supporting his wife in prayer. His awareness of God comes in the "coincidental" evidences of God's timing of things, which he finds reassuring. He recalls that it is in God that he lives and has his being, and he is concerned that his *experience* differs from this and that perhaps he is turning his back on God. Edward's assumptive world is under threat, and there is hollowness and tumult within. However, he finds some comfort in the chant that occupies "a little of the space," a prayer that the storm will be calmed and the tumult will give way to the Lord's peace.

Loss of purpose

A loved one's death may create a vacuum in what is significant, and new sources of significance, purposes, and goals must be developed.[25] For Edward now, there is little meaning in anything. His goal in those years has been to sustain his wife, and with her loss he has lost not only "half

---

25. Pargament, *Religion and Coping*, 235–39.

of himself" but also his purpose. He sees no reason to stay alive but no purpose except to maintain life, and "the future hope" does not mitigate his hopelessness. While dealing with the necessities of life, the only significant markers in this year have been the vivid weekly memories of the intimate experience of his wife's death. The fifty-second Tuesday is noted without any sense of it being a milestone to be passed. He is marking time.

Meaning-making

Meaning reconstruction is significant in mourning, and intrinsic to a person's spirituality. The journey through his wife's dementia has denied Edward the opportunity of finding meaning in the journey. The reminiscing of the family together in preparation for the funeral was a highlight for him, particularly because of his own memory difficulties. After this remembering, Edward found himself in touch with his emotions. In his sharing about the journey with the researcher, he has been quite focused on this being a contribution to benefit others on the journey, but he quite forcefully describes it as a relief, firstly that someone is listening, and secondly that it is making him "do something." Meaning needs to be made of this journey, and Edward needs opportunities to make it.

Lived Experience of Caregivers

The stories have been heard through one year of a journey of emotionally charged challenges, inevitable losses, and increasing isolation, a journey that continues indeterminately. For the person who seeks to support pastorally, drawing near to hear each story is of the essence, for if we fail to step into the world of the individual to care, we fail to care. While the experience of the individual is of ultimate concern for that person, the stories together gather power in speaking of what this all means in the wider context of care. To this drawing together and interpretation of the shared and divergent themes we now turn.

4

Caregivers' Journeys: Themes and Meanings

Almost seems like pastoral care belongs to a bygone era . . . one of the things that always concerned me is what happens to those people who've been faithful attenders at church, and suddenly . . . they can't go, and it's almost like they fall off the edge of the earth.
—Beverley

THESE STORIES GIVE US some insights into individual ongoing experiences of caregiving at different points in the journey. One caregiver participant has very recently had confirmation that it *is* the dementia journey that he and his wife have been trying to negotiate for two years. This momentous year's journey takes him from the daily pressures of trying to control the uncontrollable to a place of intense loneliness and loss, as he faces the task of rebuilding his life alone, with his distressed and confused wife in another country. Another participant travels the road a few months after the reality is named to which she has been adjusting for over two years. This year takes her from managing the relationship changes and her caregiving role with faith, friends, and a positive attitude, through a place of increasing isolation with little support or empathy, on through serious illness to a level of acceptance and the next stage of caring and letting go. Another partner is four years along the way, trying to balance caregiving with hanging on to a familiar and purposeful life. This year she moves toward a cognitive acceptance of the reality and, along with it, depression or unidentified grief. For another wife it has been a very long road, recently increasingly steep and lonely, and this year takes her further into the disenfranchised grief of family bereavement while she negotiates the daily family challenges and ongoing losses of the dementia journey. For a daughter whose life has been "on hold" for six years, this year takes her from negotiating frustrating external challenges to a somewhat better place, in spite of her mother's continuing cognitive deterioration and her own life plans still being set aside. A recently bereaved widower faces a new and darkened era, yet another chapter of the "long goodbye," a place of lonely grieving beyond which he has no incentive to move. All the travelers carry a heavy burden physically, emotionally, and spiritually, most with diminished companionship and social support. In the challenges of coping, they seek to either answer or avoid the questions of whether and where to seek help, and how to find meaning and purpose in their journey. The way ahead is of unknown duration through unchartered territory, accompanied by continuing inevitable loss.

Overall Thematic Analysis

Shared among all caregivers in the study, the overarching theme is burden, which is two-pronged, with the themes of daily functioning and ongoing loss. The sub-theme of emotional impact arises from the challenges of daily caregiving, while the sub-theme of grief lurks ambiguously in the shadow of loss. The themes of coping, meaning-making, and support emerge in response to the experiences. In the following analysis, each theme is introduced by an exemplar that compellingly captures the essence of the experience.

Burden

Daily Functioning Takes Its Toll

Exemplar:

> ELAINE: I have been a nurse . . . , but it's totally different; . . . this is 24/7, and you've got you to look after, and your partner, . . . and your house.

Six months later, after serious illness:

Caregivers' Journeys: Themes and Meanings

> ELAINE: It didn't seem to be any trouble, I was just very tired. I thought I was doing pretty well actually, but slam bang; . . . it didn't seem like a burden, but it is time-consuming, and I suppose it is wearing on your health and well-being.

Work and time pressure

For these caregivers, the practical demands are huge and exhausting. Giving care involves the time-consuming everyday challenges of maintaining the household, accommodating the loved one's memory-related limitations, and helping with personal hygiene and dressing. This is expressed succinctly:

> BEVERLEY: Basically it's all work; it's all on my shoulders; nothing happens if I don't do it.

> BEVERLEY (twelve months later): It's a bit hard when you've got to do everything—said to someone last night, "I'm sure there's a couple of hours less in each day!"

Lorraine's burden differs, in that it includes balancing the supervision of her mother's "independent" living with Lorraine's own commitments to family and work. Her caring includes the "logistic nightmare" of negotiating with medical and allied health staff during her mother's seven stays in hospital:

> Lorraine: This is my one day off, I've got to cram all this in, . . . running around trying to find nursing homes, and get interviews; . . . like, you've got to get an appointment, so then I've got to fit that around when I finish work, or I've got to start around 3 a.m. so I finish at one o'clock so that I can get these appointments. Yeah, it's frustrating in that way; . . . it's half past six, and I'm thoroughly exhausted.

Edward's experience has been different, with his wife in permanent care, but he explains that his recent months have been spent at her bedside and then being involved in making funeral arrangements, and in this experience also, there has been exhaustion.

Difficult behaviors

The deteriorating cognitive processing and functioning of their loved ones create many challenges for these caregivers. The misplacing of things and forgetting are part of the burden.

> ELAINE: He puts things away and I say, "Where did you put it?" [Colin says] "I don't know, where it belongs . . . you know where it belongs . . ." [I say] "I *don't* know where it belongs!" so we sort of go round in a circle: . . . urrggh!

The loved ones' repetitions, questions, and inability to process data place additional daily strain on the caregivers.

> BEVERLEY: If only he would stop asking questions!! Continually questioning; . . . he keeps asking . . . . Today, he's been to the dentist, she numbed his mouth. . . . He can't remember . . . *can't remember!!* . . . He says, "what did she do?" . . . I say, *"I don't know; I wasn't there!!"*

The accidents and the caregivers' necessary—but at times unwelcome—supervision of daily tasks, medications, dressing, and hygiene are demanding; and the need to supervise increases across the year. As Elaine says: "He said 'oh, look at the bathroom'; . . . he'd left the plug in and left the tap on so we had water everywhere [laugh]: . . . urgghhh." Both Henri and Lorraine have the ongoing challenge of their loved one's excessive spending, and the stress of trying to supervise this.

> HENRI: The problem is, she buys things, she can't see something without . . . she has to buy it, we don't need it, but she buys, rubbish . . . . I say *"Don't buy anything!!"* She say, "I don't buy anything!!" When she come in, she's bought a lot of stuff!!!

> LORRAINE: She just wants to spend money; she just wants, wants, wants, . . . says buying things makes her feel good. . . . So we limit, limit; . . . she gets abusive, nasty, sarcastic. I say, "Whatever."

Role changes

Four participants have the daily challenge of taking on roles formerly the province of their partner, learning to clean fish tanks, dealing with rats in the shed, and "doing everything."

Caregivers' Journeys: Themes and Meanings

> MARY: He was a very strong man, . . . always in charge, . . . someone I could count on. A role I've found very, very daunting, . . . making sure I've paid the bills, making sure his appointments were there, . . . entirely a role reversal.

Unpredictability

One element of the daily burden, referred to often, involves the unsettling and frustrating day-to-day fluctuations in the condition of their loved ones. The challenge is ongoing, as Elaine indicates: "Could get a day when everything's good—and a day when it's got a sieve in it!" Six months later, she reflects: "You get a bit frustrated, . . . 'you did it yesterday, you should do it today,' . . . but . . . it seems to be . . . random memory."

External challenges

Care for the loved one is not these caregivers' sole burden. There are other major family and personal health needs during the journey, including cancer treatment, diabetes, the death of adult children and grandchildren, increasing physical limitations and precarious health, and the long-term care of other family members. For two, their initial concerns about their partners' memory were minimized by their family doctors, and they had to push for specialist consultations. Beverley reflects: "I'd noticed twelve months before, but it took a long time for the doctor to take any notice. Couldn't get the doctor to do anything about it—brushed it off as just aging."

Emotional Impacts of Daily Burden

Exemplar:

> BEVERLEY: Afraid I take it out on him sometimes. . . . He says "you're always cranky with me." . . . I'm not cranky, just *frustrated!!* . . . Yeah, he wears it when I'm frustrated!!

Sustaining Persons, Grieving Losses

Frustration and anger

The emotional impacts of this daily burden are heard, at times loudly, in the caregivers' narratives. For the partners currently giving care, frustration and anger with the loved one are not uncommon. Beverley comments, "I don't think I'm very emotional—[I'm] fairly practical—[yet] . . . sometimes I get so angry, so frustrated, I cry!" There is divergence in Lorraine's situation; her extreme frustration early in the year emerges from her interactions with unsupportive medical and allied health staff in the hospitals.

Worry and pressure

The pressure of daily needs and demands is constant, and for all partners currently giving care, there is worry about both the present challenges and the future for their loved one. This is exemplified in Henri's experience. In the first interview, he presents a picture of constant worry: "My mind is on both sides, you know. . . . I go out, I'm worried about what she will do: . . . she can put fire in the house; . . . you have to watch her all the time, you know." Six months later, the situation is more challenging: "More pressure you know, more pressure on me, I'm scared to go out, to leave her on her own, what will happen . . . pressure, pressure, pressure all the time, you know." In the last interview, after Marguerite's relocation, the worry has not been alleviated: "When I talk to her on the phone [in Canada], I feel sad; . . . she not happy, make me worry, you know, make me worry."

Distress, disappointment, depression

Two of the caregivers take antidepressants, and a third is offered such medication during the year, as is Edward in his bereavement. Elaine voices something of the mixture of emotions expressed by all the caregiving partners. Elaine reflects, "There was anger there; . . . now, not so much anger as . . . disappointment. . . . I get upset . . . it's o.k. to get upset." A year later, she says she is coping with the daily challenges, to a degree: "most times, yes, other times I'd like to sit in a corner and bawl my eyes out." Henri also expresses a mixture of emotions: frustration, distress, turmoil and a hint of compassion mixed with a lack of understanding: "I feel sad. . . . I don't get mad, but upset. . . . I can't tell her 'you bloody mad!' you know."

Caregivers' Journeys: Themes and Meanings

Edward's experience diverges, and the daily burden of caring, feeding, and being present with his wife in her last weeks has had not only an emotional but also a spiritual impact: "I suppose... what I wrote down, was, my own spiritual life was disintegrated... in that process."

Loved ones' emotions

These caregivers also deal with other emotions, including their loved ones' anger and frustration. Lorraine, at times, is subjected to her mother's violence.

> LORRAINE: When she gets really sick... she can get really violent: ... she has punched into me, kicked me; ... just put it down to sheer frustration for her, ... not knowing who I am, or she may think I'm a stranger.

Elaine initially describes her husband as a very patient man, but six months later there are challenges: "He gets very cranky because I don't know what he's talking about; ... it's just when he can't make me understand... it's frustrating for him; it's frustrating for me!" Elaine and Beverley speak of their husbands' distress about being unable to remember, and being unable to do what they have previously done, and trying to understand or account for why they have dementia. Beverley, Elaine, and Henri refer to their partners' frustration in not being allowed to drive, forgetting that they are no longer able to. Henri has the challenge of his wife's unawareness or denial of her cognitive and functional losses, and her hostility when he tries to intervene.

Burden: Ongoing Loss Has Its Impacts

Exemplar:

> EDWARD: The long goodbye as things begin to fail—... that terminology is spot on.... [W]e started saying goodbye seven years ago; there is no reprieve, no coming back, just deterioration... you have to adapt as well as you can.

The losses and their emotional impacts are so intertwined that there is no clear distinction. Though grief is seldom identified by these caregivers, the related emotions are implicit in the many references to loss. For them, tied to the gradual but inevitable loss of the loved one as s/he has been, are the losses of relationship as it has been, and of a remembered shared past and planned shared future. The present losses are compounded by their ambiguity and by the anticipation of future losses. The caring role, by its nature, also brings loss in the caregiver's normal lifestyle and social connections. The losses have robbed three caregivers of their sense of identity.

Loved ones' losses

The awareness of ongoing deterioration is common to all participants. With it comes not just the present challenge of adjusting to the changes, but the pain of remembering what the loved one was like formerly, to which four participants refer in each of their interviews.

> ELAINE: It's terrible, . . . for what he was capable of . . . , the difference between what he was and what he is . . . , for someone so intelligent, you've got to tell him what to do—that's the hardest part; it's hard to believe.

> ELAINE (six months later): Well basically, I've lost a husband, haven't I? There's just a person there with no memory, um, basically a body, not much recollection.

> HENRI: She was very clever—she used to write a lot of poems—very, very clever, very good writer too. . . . [Now] [l]ike a child, you know, like a child . . . "Eat your food, sit down."

> MARY: He used to be strong; he used to be a group leader; . . . lots of things he's lost.

> BEVERLEY: Brain's gone, everything's gone. . . . [About playing the organ] it's gone, [faith, church connection] it's gone, . . . just gone; . . . one of the things . . . just isn't there.

> LORRAINE: Um, it was more frustrating because she had no life . . . like she was . . . not quite a vegetable, but there was no . . . nothing there, . . . she couldn't do anything. She used to do beautiful tapestry and embroidery.

Caregivers' Journeys: Themes and Meanings

All the participants recognize that the cognitive deterioration cannot be halted, but acceptance of the changes comes gradually. Edward, in retrospect, voices a sense of powerlessness and resignation.

> EDWARD: I came to accept it, because there's nothing else you can do; . . . as Evelyn's faculties or whatever terms you want to use—the mind—begins to close down and you . . . there's nothing you can do about the process, . . . it's just going to go on.

The ongoing struggle toward acceptance is expressed by Beverley. Initially, in attributing to Tom unwillingness—rather than inability—to function as previously, Beverley is intensely frustrated. A year later, she still has to remind herself regularly that he *cannot* remember: "Almost feels unreal, that a person can look so much the same, but the brain just doesn't function the same."

Loss of relational connection

All the partner participants experience a loss of companionship and a sense of isolation, and three particularly note that their partners have withdrawn into their own world.

> BEVERLEY: It makes a difference to your relationship, because you suddenly become a carer and you don't have anyone to share things with—that's hard.
>
> [And, six months later:] Oh yeah, you just feel . . . that everything's gone, yeah, nobody to talk to; . . . spend so much time at home with him, but you can't have a conversation, . . . disappointing, . . . you just feel . . . sometimes I feel like I live in an isolation bubble, . . . yeah, you know, you can't talk to him.

The loss of relationship has been devastating for Edward, who reflects on the loss that still dominates his life a year after his wife's death.

> EDWARD: Nothing can take the place of the original relationship, . . . a constant factor for the way I live now, . . . more emphasized when people are around, because the one person of significance isn't there.

For both caregiver husbands, the loss of physical closeness to their partner is very distressing. About Evelyn's move into the dementia unit of the aged care center, Edward says: "How many times we expressed love . . . , that doesn't just end, . . . to be close physically . . . a big gap not being able to be fully close." Lorraine's experience diverges markedly from the painful relational loss of the caregiver partners. Although she experiences verbal abuse, sarcasm, and occasional violence, she pragmatically sees this as her mother's failure at times to recognize Lorraine as her daughter.

Loss of emotional sharing

The sense of loss of relationship is reinforced by the absence of emotional connection, especially in times of significant loss. Mary experiences this particularly after the reappearance of their daughter's cancer.

> MARY: [I was] really, really stressed, worried, frightened. He [James] just walked past and said, "Oh well, it happens"—and just toddled off and got on the bus with his bag and off he went.

After their daughter's death, she grieves alone; her husband shows no understanding or awareness, and she is left "vulnerable, angry, um, out on my own, yeah." For Beverley, the death of their pet cat of fourteen years is difficult. When this makes no impact on her husband, she struggles with the absence of sharing in grief.

> BEVERLEY: I couldn't talk to Tom about it, he wouldn't understand; . . . well, I think I found it a bit difficult then, because there was no way I could talk about it, . . . so in one way it was good that he didn't have a reaction to the dying, but then—I'm left in limbo!

For four partners there are losses related to their family achievements and celebrations. Neither Beverley nor Elaine celebrates their wedding anniversary milestones. Elaine explains: "I thought, 'I don't want a lot of people seeing him not being what he used to be.'" Because Edward has been unable to share memories with his wife, these have faded for him. When memories are revived by his adult children in preparation for the funeral, the opportunity for reminiscence is very meaningful to him.

Loss of lifestyle

There have been major lifestyle adjustments for the caregiving partners, and a loss of shared activities and dreams of retirement. Their social connections have diminished because of time pressures, exhaustion, the circumstances of caring, and some withdrawal on the part of friends and/or

Caregivers' Journeys: Themes and Meanings

the caregivers themselves. Holidays and outings have been relinquished to varying degrees. Henri says: "I don't go out now, except Saturdays, sometimes; . . . we used to go on cruises." Lorraine's lifestyle, too, is significantly affected: "I've been sort of on hold, because of Mum." Beverley describes the caregiving experience, "I've got to live my life around caring for him," but she differs from the other partners in that, while she has relinquished some activities, she resolutely clings to others.

> BEVERLEY: I've had to give up some things; . . . I used to go to women's fellowship, and a group of retirees, but then he wouldn't come . . . I gave that up, . . . but I'm *not* giving up [a number of other community activities].

Loss of identity

Facing separation through death or relocation, both caregiving husbands see themselves, their own identity, as diminished. Edward expresses this: "It will leave a very big hole, now that half of me has died," and Henri reflects on his separation, "When she go, you've got to get used to it, you know, and that a part of me—gone!" The loss of Mary's own identity has been a long loss, and is ongoing. She thinks about this over the twelve month period:

> MARY: Sometimes I'd just like to be *Mary Kelly*, to have something for myself, knowing that it's going to get worse.

> MARY [a year later]: The things I've wanted to do have never happened, . . . it's almost as though what I wanted didn't matter. . . . [Re: setting up a counseling business:] it's something I've always wanted . . . something I've always wanted. . . . I feel that I've just been lost—[tearfully] me, myself.

On the other hand, Elaine and Beverley, still in the earlier stages of the journey, hold on to their identity in family and social roles. Lorraine, with her own family and work networks, keeps her identity intact.

Anticipatory loss

The loved ones' potential future changes cause deep anxiety; and there is awareness of the inevitability of future challenges.

BEVERLEY: I worry about him; . . . when he gets to the stage of going into care, he won't like it!

MARY: Knowing that it could get worse . . . and it's going to happen, . . . it's very upsetting. . . . [H]e made me promise I'd never put him in a situation [in a nursing home], . . . not even for respite, . . . so while he's aware . . . while things are as they are . . . .

HENRI: I don't sleep during the night, thinking about this, thinking about that, . . . what will happen.

LORRAINE: I've resigned myself that probably by the end of this year, or next year, she'll be in a nursing home; . . . yeah, it'll be the last straw kind of thing.

EDWARD: I could see what was happening, . . . that the day was coming when she'd need more care than I could do, . . . a step we knew we had to take, but it didn't make it any easier.

Across the twelve months there is anticipation of further losses.

ELAINE: It could be worse, . . . but that's into the future; . . . you know what could happen, which is sometimes rather frightening.

[Six months later:] Things could be a lot worse. . . . I know it's going to get worse, and I won't be able to manage, but at that stage, he won't know where he is or won't care where he is.

Emotional Impacts of Ongoing Loss: Unidentified Grief

Exemplar:

ELAINE [first visit]: I think there's a bit of grief. . . . I've gone through that stage. . . . [M]aybe I didn't recognize it as grief because of what I was going through; . . . it was horrendous, I suppose.

ELAINE [second visit]: Tragic, I mean you've lost your partner; . . . he's still here, but . . . and that's a bit hard to take.

ELAINE [third visit]: When someone dies it's sudden, and you accept that, but this is a gradual thing, and probably when the time comes there'll be a sigh of relief, well, he's at rest, . . . he's at peace.

Caregivers' Journeys: Themes and Meanings

Impacts of Ambiguous Loss

Grief is usually undefined, often ambiguous, and never, by their narratives, recognized or validated by others. Only Elaine refers to grief in her "living loss," but all caregiving partners readily acknowledge emotions such as sadness, anger, distress, confusion, guilt, and emptiness. The occasional, unexpected flashes of memory, insight, and lucidity bring fleeting joy—and bewilderment in the ambiguity. One particular, unexpected incident is a highlight of Mary's year.

> MARY: Well, James was always [a good speaker]—and it does come out. [W]e've been to a few things at the Center; . . . at the opening . . . he was always a very good speaker, . . . and *it's still there*. . . . He made a little speech, at the opening of the garden, . . . and . . . he was able to notice the birds coming down to the flowers and things around him, put them into the speech, . . . and it was a beautiful speech he made . . . so that part's *still there!* Oh very proud . . . and surprised—like, I nearly died when he said "oh, is it ok if I say something?" and then he went into it . . . yes . . . . But it is good to know that there is some part of him still there!

Edward, who likes to be logical in planning and preparation, has found the uncertainty of loss challenging: "I tried to think ahead and tried to work out what the various stages would be—but it's always been something different from what I expected." He, too, has been taken by surprise by his wife's occasional lucid responses. Not long before her death, when she responded verbally to the offer of Holy Communion, he was delighted: "In a sense, it was reassuring that she had something . . . that was within her. . . . She hadn't lost that!"

The grief of Henri's ambiguous loss diverges from the others' current experience, but may characterize the anticipated separation of a loved one's move into a residential aged care center. Before Marguerite leaves, he suppresses his grief: "I say, 'For your own good, you know.' I don't say I'll miss her, because I don't want to make it worse for her, so I say 'you'll be alright.'" After her move, he faces the ambiguity of her physical absence and her psychological presence. In the last interview, he speaks of the loss.

> HENRI: You've got your friend, your husband, wife, near you, and suddenly the person is gone; that's a big gap . . . you call, you call, you feel she's around, but she not here, you know; that will take time before . . . have to forget.

Edward gives insight into his post-death grief, made no easier by the years of ambiguous loss and unacknowledged grief. Shortly after her death he says, "In a sense, it was a relief." He states that now is the time for grieving, and seeks to approach the process cognitively: "Grief comes when you know it's the end; . . . in the cold light of day I can think logically about it and follow through on the progression of the parting." Twelve months later, there are "no aspirations for the remaining part of my life," and Edward reflects that his emotions have caught up with him. It has taken him a year to discover the buried grief.

Coping

Exemplar:

> ELAINE: Oh yeah, we have a few tears and a few prayers and um . . . get by . . . but even with that, there are still some good moments.

This exemplar indicates the employment of cognitive, emotional, and spiritual coping mechanisms simultaneously. Cognitive strategies vary among the caregivers, healthy expression of emotions is a regulator for several (though opportunities are limited), and spiritual practices are employed by all participants.

COGNITIVE COPING

Cognitive strategies are employed to varying degrees. Mary daily seeks to live by the Serenity prayer, mainly trying to accept what she cannot change, and once during the year, trying to change her circumstances. Elaine and Lorraine often use positive appraisals and self-talk. Henri struggles to take control of his thinking. Beverley, after her year (and more) of frustration, tries to reframe her husband's behaviors as beyond his control, rather than reacting to what she has interpreted as a lack of cooperation.

> BEVERLEY: The biggest challenge is just coping with it, just remembering that he *doesn't* remember, . . . you know, *simply doesn't!* . . . Doesn't remember, no memory—it's hard to get it through *my* brain that he really *doesn't remember!*

Cognitive control over the emotions is important to Edward, in the interviews and in life generally. He reflects, "I've always had that kind of feeling... that you can control your own life, and in the kind of emotional situation, relationships and that sort of thing"; but this experience challenges that assumption.

Affective coping

Some cry. For Beverley, who sees herself as unemotional, crying is an outlet for her intense frustration. Crying in private—either under the shower or over the ironing—provides some release for Mary. Later in the year, Elaine finds expression for her grief: "Cry... that's about it... well, if I let myself get depressed about it, I'd be a lot worse than I am."

All talk. Five participants find emotional release in conversation with someone who understands. Both Elaine and Beverley have someone in a similar caring role with whom they can talk, though their caring roles and illness interfere with this. Initially, Edward mentions one friend to whom he can speak of his loneliness, but there is no further reference to this. Henri has one friend who listens, but Henri's health issues interfere with this contact. Mary has lost the daughter with whom she had formerly shared, but she looks forward to the brief daily visits of employed caregivers with whom she can have normal conversation and a laugh. Lorraine's approach is different: over the year, her dog is her sounding board, and she is happy with this. She comments cheerfully, "My dog, oh my dog, look, she gets so much:... she says [dog sounds], she sits and looks at you."

There is some laughter. While three laugh often and two chuckle occasionally as they tell their stories, this appears to be more a release of tension than from seeing any humor in their situation. Lorraine is the only one who refers to the use of humor in her caring, when she and her mother banter in conversation, and when her mother thinks Lorraine is someone else.

Hobbies and creative pursuits have previously provided an outlet for five participants, but all explain that these are at present limited or impossible. Henri loves reading, but is unable to relax and concentrate. Beverley, Elaine, and Mary love craftwork, but for all, caregiving presents a challenge. Mary say, "I like doing craft, but when James had his stroke, that's gone by the board... I used to do scrap booking but now I can't... just too tired." Lorraine finds release in wood turning, "I massacre wood, get the frustration out," but in the ten months before and for the year of interviews, her caregiving role has prevented access to this outlet. She says, "She just follows me, and I can't have her near the lathe."

Four set aside their emotions. Because Mary's grief in the loss of her first daughter almost overwhelmed her, she feels she has to set the present grief aside: "I haven't had a real good cry . . . because you've got to keep yourself going." Beverley sees no point in crying, and prefers to be practical. Lorraine's coping is achieved by putting her emotions "on the backburner" until later.

> LORRAINE: Doesn't do anything to brood about it, it doesn't change: . . . you deal with the problem, you don't get upset, you don't get emotional, because that's where things go wrong, . . . so, like, the emotions go to the background, the practical come to the forefront.

For Edward, too, in the first interview, if emotions surface they must be put away to be dealt with privately, and he does not allow himself to be angry. Six months later, about the emotional impact of his grief Edward says with a gentle laugh, "Well, I've put that on the back burner, um, I'm dealing with everyday things." On the last visit, however, he suggests that his emotions have caught up with him.

Spiritual coping

Life principles and philosophical statements are repeated often by participants across the year, and appear to be a significant stabilizer in a destabilizing journey.

> ELAINE: You live one day at a time . . . and take it as it comes; . . . if you've got a job to do, you do it to the best of your ability.

> LORRAINE: Frustrating, because every day she hates something . . . so you *just go with the flow*.

> BEVERLEY: Just something you've got to live with. . . . I haven't blamed God . . . not that sort of person.

> HENRI: I do my best, you know, I can't do more than that . . . you have to cope, you know, there's no way round it.

> EDWARD: This is how it is, and this is how it's going to be, the acceptance of that.

Caregivers' Journeys: Themes and Meanings

> MARY: I've clung to it [the Serenity Prayer] . . . find that I'm coming up against something, I say that . . . and I seem to be able to settle myself down and look at things.

Though their understanding of spirituality varies, all participants are sustained in their journey by spiritual practices. All seek strength beyond themselves.

> LORRAINE: Never been to church on a regular basis; . . . I have my own religious beliefs. Have quiet times, sort of have a quiet word, you've got to have something to believe in, otherwise you'd just . . . probably collapse. That is a strength behind . . . got to believe in something.

The approaches to spiritual practices vary. Edward finds that the repetition of a couple of chants calms him and "fills some of the space," while for Beverley, corporate prayer is significant. Lorraine needs her quiet times to gain strength, and Henri prays for his wife and himself. Elaine reflects: "Prayer fits in, and in the middle of the frustrations . . . you think, oh, you know Lord, I'm doing the best to . . . just help me." In spite of the importance to Mary of public worship—"I find . . . faith, when I go to Mass"—and the fact that by the end of the year she can no longer attend Mass, her faith still sustains her: "I don't think it's got any less . . . it's helping me . . . I know that the power . . . ." She prays the Serenity Prayer every day and "takes strength from that."

Corporate worship is accessed by four participants, but limitations in the support received there are noted. Mary initially explains that, in attending Mass, she finds strength to face the week; later, without opportunity to attend public worship, she finds strength in social contacts. After these have also disappeared, she seeks help from her church to attend Mass, only to be disappointed. For Henri and Edward, because of their impaired hearing there is significant frustration in attending church services. Edward reflects on this: "Going to a structured form of worship, I have difficulty in hearing, so I can't hear what people are saying . . . almost makes me wonder, if I'm not finding that helpful, what do I do?"

For some, the journey has impacted on their faith. Across the year Beverley moves from never missing attending church, to finding excuses, to wondering whether she would be missed if she "dropped out." It is an effort to attend, and she does not find the services encouraging. Edward suggests that the caring journey has diminished his faith; and after his year of grieving his only hope is "the future hope" which at present does not sustain him. However, he is still able to see God's working in seeming coincidences, and to respond "Oh, You're still there!" For Henri there is a shift across the year. On the first visit he says, "God keeps me going . . . that's the purpose, you know, to look after someone." Six months later he is less confident: "I think God keeps me going . . . I don't know, I fight . . . you have to fight to survive." In his last interview, God is not mentioned.

Support

Exemplar:

> EDWARD: Unless you are experiencing it yourself, right up close, people can't understand what it's like. They say "how are you today?" and never stop long enough for . . . don't wait long enough for an answer; . . . in fact, they don't *want* an answer, don't know how to hear.

GENERAL SUPPORT

Other people's indifference and lack of understanding appear to be an experience common to these caregivers. There is some commonality, also, in their experience of support. Four speak of their family being supportive in practical ways, without further detail. Henri feels quite unsupported by his family. Only Edward mentions emotional and spiritual support from family members. Elaine's own health crisis prompts more family involvement and support, but there are reservations. She says, "You just discover how much turmoil it does cause in the family when someone's got Alzheimer's disease or dementia or whatever."

Other forms of support are limited. During the year, Mary is invited by a community Health Care provider to a monthly morning tea for family caregivers and their loved ones with dementia, which she really enjoys. It is her only social outing. Lorraine receives advice and guidance from a similar source. For Elaine, her craft group is energizing as she listens to others, and after her illness she also does some talking there. Both Elaine and Beverley explain that some friends are also busy with caregiving, and are aging and facing health issues. Mary has an uplifting but brief interlude where she has weekly contact with someone else in a similar caring role,

Caregivers' Journeys: Themes and Meanings

but this support disappears because of caregiving demands. None of the participants have accessed a support group.

> BEVERLEY: Have been told there's an Alzheimer's group I can go to ... that's all that's happened. ... A few of us in the church said we ought to set up our own [support] group, but it hasn't happened!
>
> BEVERLEY (a year later): [the group] never did form, to a certain extent it's a pity, um, it's knowing what you need.

Pastoral support

None of the participants speak of ongoing support from a church community. Three have been significantly involved in their local churches for many years, and two have had previous connections with a congregation. Elaine had earlier received a few pastoral visits in which her husband was included, but these ceased with a change of church staff. Her husband has not been visited since. There have been a few pastoral encouragements. For Edward, one lady at church has listened to him "a couple of times," and her listening with empathy was meaningful for him: "a few 'bloodys' in there from her ... was great, someone's being real in the situation!" For Elaine, occasional emails from someone at church helped: "it was an awful day, and she sent me a prayer and it was wonderful, at just the right time." Mary had one visit from a community chaplain, which she appreciated because they were able to talk like friends "just about ordinary things," and she and her family received a visit from a Service Club chaplain before her daughter's funeral. She reflects on this:

> MARY: He really, really spent a lot of time with us ... you know, listened to what we were telling him about her, and I just thought ... I got more support from him than what I did from my parish priest.

Six months after the death of his wife, Edward speaks about pastoral support.

> EDWARD: Don't know whether people assume that I don't need it ... perhaps because of the fact that I have been ordained myself ... whether people think that you can pull yourself up [quiet laugh] by your own boot straps.

Six months further on, he suggests, "Perhaps I'm too difficult a character to deal with."

Henri and Mary have both formerly attended public worship—Mary, for about fifty years in the local congregation—but Mary's reduced mobility prevents attendance and Henri has become disconnected because of health and hearing issues. Participating in the sacrament of Holy Communion is important for them. For Henri, during the year a pastor friend initiates fortnightly-to-monthly home visits to share the sacrament with him and Marguerite. Mary wishes she could receive Holy Communion, but when she finally sees the priest this is not offered.

Congregational support

Beverley feels that she could withdraw from the congregation without being missed, though she has held significant positions during her many years of involvement, along with her husband, who was an organist for many years until his dementia led to his withdrawal. He has not been visited. She reflects, "The church, no, I wouldn't say they've been supportive; . . . I've got to make an effort to go, or I'd withdraw."

The contrast in the level of empathy offered in physical illness and in caring for a loved one with dementia is evidenced in the narration of two participants. Elaine feels the isolation of the dementia journey in the lack of understanding of her friends. She says, "I don't think people realize he's as bad: . . . one said to me "oh, when will he get better?" Six months later, after her own illness where she has been surrounded by warm and caring support, there is a different response, "a lot of help, lot of support . . . friends are absolutely great." Edward, having watched the support offered to someone who had had a heart attack, notes the difference in response.

> EDWARD: You've got something there that people expect people to talk about; . . . people can say, "oh, I'm sorry about that" or "it must be difficult for you" . . . talk about it quite clearly and know what they're meaning . . .
>
> INTERVIEWER: People support them?
>
> EDWARD: All the time, and put their arm around them, . . . but ah, it's an embarrassment when you're dealing with the personality and what's happening there; . . . people find it embarrassing, and they don't know how to deal with it . . . .

Caregivers' Journeys: Themes and Meanings

INTERVIEWER: And what effect does that have on you?

EDWARD: Oh, you're in an empty space....

Desired support

Each participant is invited to suggest what emotional or spiritual support might be helpful. Lorraine has no suggestions; she has not thought about support. Among the others, there is unanimity about the need to be heard, but for some this gives way to ambivalence and a strong thread of doubt in light of their experiences.

> HENRI (without hesitation): To talk about it, it's good, if you have somebody to talk to, ... but somebody who [will] understand....
> But some people you can't talk [to] about it; they don't understand.
> ... I can't even talk to my daughter or son.
>
> (six months later): Nobody to talk to, nobody, and ah, it's difficult to talk, you know, people should understand but they don't understand: ... "Dad will be alright" ... but I'm *not* alright!

Initially Elaine speaks of the desire to talk to someone who understands: "Just someone to come and visit ... talk to me, listen to me ..."; but six months later, when her friends have failed to understand, she is not so sure: "I don't know, it could help, having someone to talk to, but if they're not in that situation they don't really understand."

As well as the need to be understood, two participants express the desire for listening to be complemented by prayer. Having reflected on people not wanting to hear him, Edward knows what support he would like: "Oh, being able to listen, and then support in prayer; ... to listen and take up what you've been talking about, so that you feel you've got something out of it." Beverley regrets the absence of corporate prayer for the personal needs of congregation members.

Help-seeking

Exemplar:

> MARY: You're asking for help ... I've been able to do it without help before ... I suppose it's me realizing that it's me not coping now ... yes, not coping ... a sign of weakness.

The exemplar reflects something the struggle common to these caregivers in asking for help. Three are reluctant, seeing this as an indication of not coping, or of imposing on others, or of acknowledging the next stage of the journey. Two do not know what would help or what support is available. Edward thinks it is expected that he will not need help, and he does not seek it. So during the year the "next stage" of support is thrust upon Elaine after her serious illness; anti-depressants are offered to—and refused by—Edward and Beverley; Henri relinquishes Marguerite's care to her daughter in Canada; and Lorraine is frustrated in trying to access information about practical support. She reflects, "If you don't know what to ask for or what you're entitled to, no one will help you." Beverley, who across the year has experienced intense frustration and then some depression, does not know what would help: "yeah, if you don't know what to look for." A year later she explains her reluctance:

> BEVERLEY: To a certain extent, if the church is going to do something for you, somebody's got to put themselves out . . . haven't really expected that other people should put themselves out.

For Henri, in the last interview there is a sense of hopelessness as he faces life alone, and there is no help: "I don't know what to do, you know, I need help, but I don't know what door to knock."

Only Mary finally seeks emotional and spiritual support. It takes the death of her second daughter for her to overcome her great reluctance. She is offered nothing but platitudes from the priest: "Oh, you know, I'll see them in heaven, and it's God's will, and um, I didn't want that . . . so I just haven't bothered." When she in desperation speaks to her family doctor, he is not interested in her, preferring to talk about how her husband is, and this gentle lady says, "I just, I got really angry . . . I did, I left the surgery!"

Meaning-making

Exemplar:

> EDWARD: One has to accept it . . . an imperfect world . . . in our humanity, there are imperfections . . . no answers to the question "why?" . . . not this side of the grave.

Caregivers' Journeys: Themes and Meanings

Making sense

Approaches to making meaning in the journey vary. Some look for reasons, but find any explanation elusive. Beverley wonders whether an accident that happened years earlier contributed to her husband's condition, or whether her husband has not exercised his brain enough. By the last interview, she still wishes for some answers, but no longer blames her husband for his condition, taking a more positive approach: "this is the way it pans out, so try and make the best of it." Elaine also wonders why, but she finds meaning in making the best of it.

> ELAINE: You feel he didn't deserve that, . . . we did all the right things; . . . they say to keep your mind active. . . . I get upset . . . unfairness about why it happened. . . . You don't [try to make sense of it], you just go with the flow, and think you're not the only one; . . . you don't get angry with God.

Henri is initially cheerfully pragmatic: "Oh, that's life, my dear, life is not a bed of roses . . . up and down, you know, sometimes more down than up; . . . you can't win all the time, you know." Later in the year, the pragmatism is replaced by a sense of life's meaninglessness.

Finding meaning and purpose

In this difficult journey, four participants find purpose in commitment to marriage and/or family.

> EDWARD: In the marriage service "the two become one" . . . and you live life on that basis, . . . and then the end . . . because of the love we had for one another . . . to be able to respond to that . . . .

> LORRAINE: [The financial adviser says] "Let her be kicked out" [of her home]. But that's not me . . . it's a family; . . . what'd I be teaching my own kids, if I do that sort of thing to my mother?

> MARY: My upbringing, . . . my grandparents, . . . everything around the family, . . . that's helped to . . . I still carry those values.

In the first interview, Henri finds meaning in caring: "You know, God keeps me going . . . that's the purpose, you know, to look after someone." A year later that purpose has been lost, and there is nothing to sustain him:

> HENRI: You're at that stage, there's nothing for you to do on this earth.... I will feel bored, I will feel lost; ... no good, no good.... I think when you reach the stage like this, they should allow you to put yourself down, the doctor should give you an injection.

Life review

Three of the participants say that they find meaning and value in sharing their story with the researcher.

> MARY: Makes me see things as they are. It's good to get it out, it's good to verbalize it because now it's real!

> MARY (twelve months later): It does help, because you're not just sitting there thinking "oh, woe is me" ... because you're bringing it out and um ... you're acknowledging ... really, what's happening and how you're feeling about things, and how it's affecting you, where if you're keeping it inside, it's not good.

> HENRI: Good to talk about it ... you have to breathe sometime ... you know, you have to breathe, let it out.... I'm more open to talk to you than my son and daughter; ... if I told my daughter, she'd say "what I can do?" That's it, she just turn the page, that leave me [he takes a deep breath, and holds it.]

> EDWARD (at the end of the last interview): A relief that somebody's listening ... and I suppose it's ... giving some relief that ... not only is somebody listening, but it's making me *do* something.

Implications for Care

What do these journeys, with their shared themes and divergent experiences, mean in the broader context of dementia care; and how do they illuminate the pastoral process for the dementia journey? These are physically and emotionally demanding, spiritually challenging, and relationally isolating journeys. These caregivers experience the burden of daily functioning with all its frustrations, responsibilities, and uncertainties; and, intertwined with the challenges, every day they are confronted by loss, inevitable, unpredictable, and sometimes unbelievable, with its often unnamed but at times devastating emotional impacts. They have limited opportunities for identifying or expressing their emotions or making sense of their experience. Two participants whose partners are in early dementia maintain some of their interests, but several have little or no time or energy for their leisure activities. Edward and Henri, left alone, have little interest in anything. Spiritual questions of the meaning of this experience in relation to their assumptive worlds are generally unasked and unanswered. There is no reference to any discussion with the loved one about negotiating present or future emotional or spiritual challenges together, or to any acknowledgment of these challenges within the family or their social context or their church. Their coping resources are stretched; and cognitive, affective, and spiritual strategies are applied with varying effectiveness. Emotional support is intermittent for most, given by friends in similarly pressured caring roles; and spiritual support is fragmentary and generally not offered. Help-seeking is avoided. Unless there are changes in their circumstances that allow them to tell their stories and make meaning in this journey, nebulous grief, existential loneliness, and spiritual pain may be their increasingly insistent companions until and beyond the death of the loved one.

Burden: Emotional Impacts

Loss and Grief

For those still giving care, the emotional impacts of the daily burden interact with the unidentified grief of their ongoing losses. The frustrations related to their loved ones' changed behavior, diminishing functioning, fraught communication, and role relinquishment are accompanied by memories of what no longer is, and fears of losses still to come. There are references in every narrative to the past qualities of the loved one, and to the uncertain certainty of what the future holds. The loss is ambiguous and confusing: the person may look the same, but is not; the person may reappear briefly as she or he was, before "disappearing" again; or the person is expected to behave as the adult she has been while being cast in the role of a naughty child. A further component of the load verbalized by three caregivers is an anticipatory concern for how their partners will feel about future losses and challenges. The caregivers' responses to the losses are generally not identified as grief, and it is frustration that is often articulated, and depression that is diagnosed.

It would appear that there is neither time nor opportunity to recognize their grief for what it is, nor are there resources available for processing it. The one caregiver who reflects on her feelings of having already lost her husband and on her anticipated relief after his death chooses not to reflect on when or how she might grieve. For the caregiving partners, the emotions do push their way out in anger, pain, sadness, confusion, guilt, chronic sorrow, and existential loneliness. It is notable that for one (Beverley), the gradual acceptance of the reality of her partner's cognitive losses during the year coincides with increasing episodes of what she and her family doctor describe as depression, and it is also interesting that four at least have been offered antidepressants. For the bereaved partner, the present grief is not mitigated by the "long goodbye" that has been. It takes a year for him to experience the emotions, and in his grief he is offered antidepressants.

The major contribution of grief to caregiver burden has recently been highlighted in dementia studies.[1] Where there is pervasive sadness or desperation in undefined long-term loss, opportunities should be provided for gaining insight into the grief and for reconstructing meaning.[2] In their isolation from the normal flow of life, both of the long-term caregivers (Mary for over twenty years and Edward for seven years) experience chronic sorrow and existential loneliness; and both indicate that sharing their story has been valuable in discovering and processing their emotions. The ambiguous and ongoing loss articulated by all the caregiving partners is a heavy load borne alone, with little opportunity to explore their emotions or have their experience normalized. Their grief is generally not recognized by themselves or their families or professionals, and evidently not acknowledged in their wider networks and church contexts. If their grief were identified and supported by appropriate interventions, the isolation and distress of the journey might be reduced. If grief interventions *per se* were offered, it is doubtful whether these caregivers would accept them because of the undefined nature of their grief. In telling their stories, however, the losses are identified and the grief work is undertaken.

Along with their other losses, several partners are losing a sense of who they are personally. Personal goals are important in creating meaning, but several of the caregivers have set these aside. For two, the demands of caring have hijacked their personal goals and cut off their external connections, their social network, and their church; and there is a sense of having

---

1. See chapter 5 for an exploration of grief.
2. Neimeyer and Jordan, "Disenfranchisement," 105–8.

lost who they were. Two caregivers who are early in the journey still cling to their social context and meaningful social roles, and maintain a personal identity. Both anticipate losses ahead, their connections diminish during the year, and the nebulous loss of their planned couple future separates them from friends in their cohort. Three partners express the belief that other people are embarrassed by dementia and avoid conversation; and the sense that their journey cannot be understood by others deprives them of emotional connection and recognition of their caregiving. Indeed, there is no indication of any affirmation of their caregiving role, or opportunity of integrating their caregiving into their identity.

It is generally recognized that couples build a shared social identity; and with the losses of the dementia journey, this shared identity needs to be renegotiated and reconstructed. Challenges to couple-identity for these caregivers include losses such as attending church services with their partner, celebrating significant milestones and sharing pride in family achievements, sharing the grief of significant family losses, remembering their common past, and, of course, facing their unknown future. Shared activities are lost, and although two caregivers persevere with couple outings, these cannot be remembered together afterwards. Though at least one couple has been part of a friendship network of couples, they are no longer involved. Three caregivers feel that their partners have retreated into their own world, and they feel a loss of intimacy and companionship and a deep sense of isolation. It is interesting to note that for Mary, couple-identity is fostered when a monthly morning tea is instituted for caregivers and their loved ones with dementia; and it is here that she experiences deep pride and joy in seeing something of her husband's former self. The loss of couple-identity has begun years earlier for Edward with his wife's move into permanent care; but this loss is not grieved until her death severs, as he sees it, half of him. With the relocation of Henri's wife, the loss of couple-identity is ambiguous: he is still married, but alone; he is free of the stresses of caring, but agonizes in the loneliness of separation and the challenge of rebuilding his life. Such ambiguous loss of couple-identity is faced in anticipation, and then in reality, by caregivers who place their partner in permanent care. Edward, Henri, and indeed all caregiving partners whose loss of shared identity is slow and ambiguous, are presented with questions of adjustment and reconstruction of identity.

Sustaining Persons, Grieving Losses

Identity and Meaning-making

Meaning-making involves reconstructing a new way of being-in-the-world, and a new sense of identity out of one's former sense of self; and this process is especially important in complicated grief.[3] Conversations open the way for building self-identity and integrating new meaning in the identity. Because of their burden, their diminishing social world, and their sense that other people cannot understand their journey, these caregivers do not generally engage in narrative processes that might allow them to review their experience or reconstruct their identity. For the two caregivers facing the loss of their wives, there are limited opportunities to tell their story, rebuild their lost identity, make sense of their experience, or find new purposes to replace their former purpose of caregiving. In the absence of a context for telling her story, Mary, whose caregiving has spanned more than two decades, feels that her own identity has already been lost and there are no remaining purposes other than caregiving.

Long-term loss and bereavement present a crisis in meaning, and sense needs to be made early in the experience. It may be deeply distressing if a significant event or loss cannot be readily assimilated into a person's assumptive world. What will not fit the belief system may be ignored, or the belief system may be accommodated in a new framework. These caregivers indicate some of the values of their assumptive worlds: if we do the right things, all will be well; everything can be dealt with logically with the emotions under control; God's purpose is for me to give care; the church is always right; you can push through the difficulties and they will pass; the emotions can be put aside; there is no place for anger toward God. Their journeys challenge these beliefs. Their global meaning systems are confronted by different situational meanings, and the differences are difficult to ignore.

Meaning-making is difficult in their situations; and several say, "You don't make sense of it." Because loss presents a crisis in meaning, sense needs to be made of the loss for it to be assimilated into the existing belief system, or the belief system accommodated in a new framework.[4] There is no social or spiritual environment where the situational meaning of their daily experience can be reappraised or where disparity between global meaning and situational meaning can be identified and negotiated.

---

3. Neimeyer and Currier, "Bereavement Interventions," 18.
4. Neimeyer and Anderson, "Meaning Reconstruction Theory," 48–49.

CAREGIVERS' JOURNEYS: THEMES AND MEANINGS

Nonetheless, these caregivers find meaning in values that give a sense of purpose, in ongoing commitment and love, and in a task to be accomplished to the best of their ability. The major personal goal verbalized by five caregivers is, or has been, to give their loved one the best possible care. Where there is no opportunity to define the caregiving role or integrate it into the overall narrative and the self-identity, there may be a sense of lost identity or wasted ("on hold") life. On the other hand, where this goal of caregiving becomes paramount and meaning is not found beyond this purpose, where identity is not nurtured, where the network fails, and where the spiritual life is not sustained in community, it is unsurprising that the loss of the caring role and the loved one's death present a crisis. As the meaningful task of caring ceases for two partners, they lose their sense of purpose and see little or no point in living.

If, in the years of caregiving, people are not given ongoing opportunities for integrating the meaning of the journey into their assumptive worlds and life purposes, what does remain for them following the death of their loved one? The story needs to be heard, again and again, and with deep empathy. If it is heard throughout the journey, this experience may become a meaningful part of a larger life story of a person who loves and a loved one who is loved, of persons whose identities have been sustained and enriched by the experience. If not, an emptiness around and hollowness within, an existential loneliness, may be the bitter fruit of this journey.

Empathic conversation encourages a social processing that helps grievers to realize and accept losses, and invites them to make sense of the experience or at least to find some positive aspects if sense-making is not possible. In talking, Mary sees that her experience of the grief journey is "real"; Beverley gradually processes and moves toward acceptance of her husband's cognitive losses; Henri voices the anticipatory grief that he has concealed for Marguerite's sake; Lorraine relaxes; Elaine begins to explore her grief; Edward discovers his emotions and finds himself "doing something" with the experience; and all reminisce on significant elements of their loved one's identity.

Social interventions are advocated, both to support caregivers in dealing with relational deprivation and loss of self, and to support the caregiver and the person with dementia together in negotiating these challenges.[5] For these caregivers and their loved ones, shared negotiation of meaning and validation of their emotions early in the journey might have facilitated

5. Adams et al., "Personal Losses," 313–16.

ongoing meaning-making in what might otherwise become stressful chaos or meaningless existence, during their journey and beyond. Four participants verbalize the value and/or the relief of telling their story to the researcher, and all communicate a positive response in their narratives and body language. In the ambiguity of the losses, through sharing their story they begin to discover what is lost that needs to be grieved, and what is still there that can be sustained, nurtured, and enhanced.

Empathic Failure

For these six caregivers, opportunities for such processing have been minimal. While several acknowledge the value of empathic listening, their experience suggests that this is available only from other caregivers; but these stories highlight the precarious nature of such support, with increasing caregiving demands and the vulnerable health of caregiving friends. The empathic failure in their networks, including their churches, during this ambiguous and long grief calls for attention. (It is interesting that one sees her dog as an empathic listener!) If supportive social and/or spiritual networks are to be maintained around both caregivers and persons with dementia, a broader understanding of dementia and the challenges and opportunities of the journey is urgently needed. Initiatives for support need to come from other people, for help-seeking does not come easily, and in the midst of the challenges it is difficult to know "on which door to knock."

Meaning-making: A Spiritual Process

Meaning-making is recognized as a spiritual task, and faith or spirituality may provide a theoretical construct for making sense of this journey. All of these caregivers see their experience in spiritual terms, ranging from receiving the strength to cope from something beyond, through drawing on a personal faith and talking to God, to the perceived disintegration of the spiritual life. For three, there is a profound sense of disconnectedness within and/or without, and an existential loneliness or emptiness. Spirituality relates to feeling integrated and connected. Where connection, purpose, and hope have been lost and situational meaning cannot be reconciled with global meaning, and where there is no opportunity for making meaning or finding purpose, spiritual pain prevails. For these people, making sense of this journey and easing their pain will not be achieved by a course of anti-depressants; rather, this is a spiritual journey to be traveled in company with others who permit them to voice, and make sense of, their spiritual questions.

Coping

For these caregivers, this is a journey where ongoing ambiguous losses, exhaustion, constant communication problems, and unpredictable changes put pressure on cognitive and affective coping strategies. They employ positive self-talk to varying degrees, in narrating and analyzing the situation. However, day to day there is little opportunity to verbalize positive appraisals of the situation. The employment of coping strategies to regulate affect is limited, and emotions are expressed alone in private, shelved, or directed at the person with dementia or others. It is a testimony to the determined resilience of these people that they have coped thus far with the multi-faceted challenges in caregiving.

There are quite wide-ranging approaches to spirituality among these participants, but all employ religious and/or spiritual strategies in coping with the demands of caregiving. The contribution of spirituality or faith is conceived by them in a variety of ways: to gain strength, wisdom, patience, and calm in the midst of turmoil, to connect with a power beyond, and to give purpose. All of these caregivers pray, and the longing is expressed by three for someone else to pray for or with them. Having a voice is an important way of maintaining identity in aging, and prayer is a powerful means of having a voice, of sustaining identity and faith, and of creating meaning and discerning purpose in life.[6] Although they do not generally feel heard by others, and although meaning and purpose may not be easy (or possible) to discern, prayer is significant.

For three of these caregivers, faith in God is acknowledged to be intrinsic to the daily journey. The Scriptures, congregations, and a person's spiritual experiences and religious beliefs may come together to provide a system of religious support that individuals can draw on in their efforts to sustain themselves in the midst of turmoil and change.[7] While these caregivers express the need to individually reach beyond themselves toward the transcendent, they appear to have little expectation or experience of support from the Christian community, and there are few references to

6. Eisenhandler, *Keeping Faith*, 94–96.
7. Pargament, *Religion and Coping*, 212.

the Scriptures. There is little indication of encouragement in their faith journeys from within congregations, through corporate worship, by others' prayer, or by their church leaders.

Support

"Thin" Support

Emotional and spiritual support from beyond their family/friendship networks has been generally absent. For many people in the older cohort, the religious community is recognized as an important source of support.[8] It is notable that for the three caregiving partners who have been closely involved in serving their church community for many years, such support is apparently minimal, though one receives warm support during physical illness. For two previously connected with churches, there has been almost no support.

Diminution of friendship support is common to the caregiving partners in this study. This is attributed to several factors: the inhospitable behavior of the person with dementia toward the caregiver's friends, the aging cohort's health issues, others' busyness with life and church affairs, embarrassment and a lack of understanding of dementia, and unwillingness to listen, with the consequent withdrawal of caregivers. The contrast of the support given to church members with physical illness is wistfully noted by one person, while another accepts the contrast without question, appreciating what is offered in her serious physical illness. While two of the loved ones with dementia are supported by external networks (for one, sustained involvement in service groups, and for the other, initially, a church-related small group), their caregivers are isolated at home and receive little social support. (However, later in the year, one of these caregivers greatly values a monthly social event organized by a community service provider for persons with dementia and caregivers.)

Help-seeking Reluctance

The attitudes toward help-seeking expressed by these caregivers reflect those of a society that places a high value on personal independence. The

---

8. Settersten, "Sources of Meaning," 61–62.

reluctance to ask for help arises from several sources: the perception that asking for help equates to weakness and a failure to cope; an unwillingness to acknowledge "the next stage" that might not be negotiable alone; the absence of expectation of emotional or spiritual support; the assumption that others are too busy to help; and the unwillingness to impose on others. It is noteworthy that there are no different expectations of care or support from the churches represented than from anywhere else—and on the one occasion when, in desperation, help is finally sought from the church community, the damaging response more than confirms Mary's expectations and reinforces her reluctance. If appropriate support is to be provided in this journey in this culture, it may not be because caregivers ask.

The Journey

While it is not valid to generalize conclusions from a very small group of caregivers, each story gives insight into the challenges of caring for a loved one with dementia; and together they broaden the understanding of the emotional and spiritual needs of caregivers. As described by this diverse group at different stages of caregiving, this is a journey attended by (usually unidentified) grief. It is, for several, an isolating, lonely journey, a tough road, "narrow, very narrow," as they experience a gradual loss of their loved ones as they have known them, their relationship and life as it has been, and to varying extents, connection with their friends and networks. For the caregiving partners the loss is major, and the emotions are intense. Coping resources, so central to how the journey is negotiated, are stretched at times to the limit. As these resources are depleted, the effects feed back into greater burden, stress, loss, and emotional and physical vulnerability, which in turn create a less supportive environment for their loved ones with dementia. If the resources are to be strengthened, if the caregivers' lives and the lives of their loved ones are to be sustained, if grief is to be processed, help from beyond themselves is called for.

5

Grieving Losses: "The Long Goodbye"

Give sorrow words. The grief that does not speak whispers the fraught heart, and bids it break.
—MACBETH, ACT 4, SC 3

AMONG THE MANY CHALLENGES of the dementia journey, there is, then, the question of what to do with the losses. There is an extremely strong case for fighting against a malignant social positioning of a person as a lost self or an empty shell, through telling a larger story of a valued person whose personhood remains undiminished; but there is also another pressing reality, the ongoing reality of loss. Early in dementia, persons with dementia are cognitively aware of losses, present and anticipated, articulated or ignored; and there is no reason to doubt that later, often without the capacity for verbal expression, a person continues to *emotionally* experience losses. Throughout a family caregiver's journey, while it is crucial for the caregiver to relate to and love the present person and to sustain his/her identity, there are ongoing losses that cannot be ignored, and in the loved one's death, there is more loss. And where there is loss, there is grief.

In recent years there has been an increasing awareness of the impact of grief on the well-being of those facing the challenges of dementia. While research seeks to untangle the realities of this particular grief, there are still gaps in understanding and a general absence of interventions to address its impacts. There have been few attempts to relate bereavement theories to the often long pre-death losses, and fewer to consider to what extent these theories are relevant to caregivers' complex post-death experience.

A brief overview of recent bereavement grief theories and of recent dementia research gives a context for identifying the challenges in the losses that caregivers face, both before and after the death of a person with dementia. As research and theoretical developments gradually illuminate the issues, a framework is needed for effective interventions. After considering the challenges, a spiritual framework is found to be appropriate, wherein support may be offered to both caregivers and persons with dementia in making meaning in the grief, addressing the pain, sustaining the identity, nurturing the person, transcending the loss, and enhancing well-being through the journey and into caregivers' bereavement. Such a framework also offers opportunities and challenge to the Christian community to support those on this faith journey in churches and to reach out to the broader community to offer loving, compassionate care in the name of Christ.

Bereavement Grief

Theories

Single Pathway Models

"Single pathway" theories elaborate tasks and processes of grieving and moving on through bereavement. An influential model describes "tasks of mourning" that vary in difficulty for different mourners.[1] These tasks, that may need to be renegotiated over time, include accepting the reality, irreversibility, and meaning of the loss; processing rather than avoiding the pain; adjusting to the environment without the deceased person; adjusting the belief system and the sense of self in the world; and embarking on a new life, making space for other relationships through relocating rather than relinquishing the deceased.[2] Rando's model also describes sequential phases of mourning: avoidance, where the challenge is to acknowledge the death; confrontation, where the pain of the loss is experienced and the relationship as it has been is relinquished; and accommodation, where the bond is maintained through healthily relocating the deceased as a reference point.[3]

---

1. Worden, *Grief Counseling*, 27–29.
2. Ibid., 29–37.
3. Rando, *Complicated Mourning*, 30–43.

Thus the mourner moves on in life and invests in other relationships. However, Rando notes that long illness, stress, and lack of social support may impede such processing and contribute to complicated post-death grief.[4]

Dual Process Model

Other recent theories, rather than presenting sequential steps to recovery, propose that the processes of experiencing the pain of loss and adjusting the sense of self and the world occur concurrently during the grieving. The dual process model presents the grief process as an oscillation between a *Loss* orientation, where the pain of grief is experienced and the relationship is restructured internally, and a *Restoration* orientation, where attention is directed outward toward reentering life and rebuilding new relationships; and healthy bereavement grieving is indicated where the loss orientation decreases with time, and the outward and forward orientation becomes more pervasive.[5]

Continuing Bonds Theory

A "continuing bonds" perspective argues that the grief process involves a symbolic mental relocation of the deceased person to a comforting background presence that provides a secure base for the bereaved.[6] Field's work builds on this, identifying processes of *deconstruction*—through becoming aware in different contexts that the deceased is dead, and along with the deceased, the related hopes, plans, and expectations—and *reconstruction*, a cognitive restructuring that, while acknowledging the affective pain, produces a new meaningful life where the bond continues internally.[7] A coherent narrative of this loss is constructed within the context of the larger life story.[8] These theories deal with a clear-cut loss through bereavement, with the goal of moving on in life through cognitively processing the loss and relocating the deceased person as a background presence.

---

4. Ibid., 297–301.
5. Stroebe and Schut, "Dual Process Model," 5–8.
6. Silverman and Nickman, "Concluding Thoughts," 349–53.
7. Field, "Relinquish or Maintain," 86.
8. Field and Wogrin, "Unresolved Loss," 38–39.

Grieving Losses: "The Long Goodbye"

Meaning-making Theory

A recent approach presents meaning reconstruction as the core element in bereavement grieving. Neimeyer maintains that in the disruption of personal identity and the crisis of meaning precipitated by the death of a loved one, the central tasks of grieving include: acknowledging the emotional responses; making meaning in the loss; and rebuilding the identity and place in the world through a self-narrative that incorporates the loss.[9] Because the loss of a central figure in the bereaved person's life story seriously disrupts her self-narrative, the task becomes the cognitive development of a new sense of self in the absence of the deceased, in a self-narrative that incorporates the loss through an internal acknowledgment of emotional responses, a reflexive process of analyzing what the loss means, and a social text.[10] Such a process is associated with reduced symptoms in bereavement; and complicated grief is indicated where these tasks are not completed.[11] Where there is a profound discrepancy between the person's assumptive world—the person's taken-for-granted narratives and values—and the present experience, the search for meaning in the loss may be unsatisfied; and where there has been a lack of coherence in the mourner's identity over time, the reconstruction of identity and a new self-narrative may be impeded.[12]

While these tasks of personal meaning-making and reconstruction of the self-narrative are central in grieving, the importance of the social context and social processes must not be overlooked. In fact, Walter argues that bereavement behavior is driven by the need to make sense of the self and others, through narrative with others who knew the loved one,[13] and Gillies and Neimeyer claim that "our lives, our identities and our meaning structures are social constructions, a web of connections created through our ongoing discourse with the social world in which we live."[14] Neimeyer explains the grief process as an oscillation between internal meaning-making and this social processing.[15] An individual's bereavement grief is

---

9. Neimeyer, *Meaning Reconstruction*, 2–4.
10. Neimeyer and Anderson, "Meaning Reconstruction Theory," 51–54.
11. Neimeyer, "Language of Loss," 263–66.
12. Shear et al., "Complicated Grief," 144.
13. Walter, "Bereavement and Biography," 19–20.
14. Gillies and Neimeyer, "Search for Significance," 61.
15. Neimeyer, "Language of Loss," 266–68.

usually experienced within the family system, and its social processing will be related to both the level of cohesion and emotional expression within the family network, and to the deceased person's role within that network.[16] Within the family system, grief processing may be facilitated through empathic encouragement and sharing of emotions, and through reminiscing, helpful in sustaining the identity of the griever.[17] Shared meanings within the family are fostered by mourning rituals, which are beneficial in acknowledging the changed status of the bereaved, for example from wife to widow.[18] The social process of grieving and moving on may be facilitated through constructing a biography, preferably with family members or others with shared understandings of the person, but failing this, in a self-help bereavement group with people who have experienced loss of a similar kind and share similar feelings.[19]

The social process facilitates validation of the self, new patterns of functioning, and the rebuilding of a place in the world; and supportive relationships in the social environment contribute to resilience.[20] Obviously, difficulties in processing may be exacerbated by grievers' withdrawal from their social world, or by the withdrawal, either physical or emotional, of others in the family or social world. For some time it has been recognized that narrative, facilitated by an empathic companion, is an important component of healing in losses, as a way of finding meaning and purpose and a new way of living and being.[21] Such a supportive listener, external to the family, might journey with the bereaved person, and through deep listening and conversation, allow the person to negotiate the meaning of the loss, reorganize the connection with the deceased, and reconstruct the disrupted self-identity and self-narrative.[22] On reflection, it is evident that such bereavement processes are not readily applied where much loss has occurred before death, particularly where the social network is no longer available, where family cohesion has been compromised, and where the griever's life narrative has been disrupted over a long period of unacknowledged loss.

16. Worden, *Grief Counseling*, 150–58.
17. Ibid., 168.
18. Neimeyer et al., "Mourning and Meaning," 236.
19. Walter, "Bereavement and Biography," 15–19.
20. Ibid., 23.
21. Neimeyer and Gamino, "Grief and Bereavement," 851.
22. Neimeyer and Jordan, "Disenfranchisement," 109.

Complicated Grief

Disenfranchised Grief

The absence of acknowledgment and support in a loss gives rise to disenfranchised grief, where "there is no social recognition that the person has a right to grieve or a claim for social sympathy or support."[23] The lack of validation of grief, or "empathic failure," may occur not only in bereavement but in such situations as "social death" where a living person is treated as dead, or "psychosocial death" where a person has changed and is not related to as the same person.[24] Such disenfranchisement of grief and empathic failure are likely to be the experience of the primary caregiver of a person with dementia, and the person with memory loss herself, where there may be an absence of support in the multiple losses over a number of years.[25]

Ambiguous Loss

In losses where the boundaries are blurred between what is lost and what is not lost, the impacts of grief are significant. For example, where a person is physically present but psychologically absent, or is psychologically present but physically absent, the loss is ambiguous, and grieving is complex and immobilizing.[26] In such situations the person may be treated by some members of the family as wholly present and by others as wholly absent, with ensuing personal and interpersonal stress and conflict within the family; and the impacts of such ambiguity are likely to be a sense of helplessness, anxiety, and depression.[27] Episodes of lucidity even into advanced dementia may increase the ambiguity and the emotional impact on family members, possibly serving as cruel reminders of the past, or as signs of hope.[28] The ambivalence of conflicted emotions, of hope and grief for example, may not be resolvable; and if the ambiguity and ambivalence are not normalized, the outcomes may be guilt, unresolved grief, and paralyzing

---

23. Doka, "Disenfranchised Grief," 224.
24. Ibid., 224–26.
25. Doka, "Grief and Dementia," 145–50.
26. Boss, *Loss, Trauma*, 7–12.
27. Ibid., 38.
28. Killick and Allan, *Communication*, 274–75.

stress in relationships.[29] Boss argues that the most important predictor of resilience is the ability to hold two opposing ideas at the same time, being flexible and able to live comfortably with ambiguity and unanswered questions.[30] In addressing ambiguous loss, an appropriate intervention may support a griever by assisting in naming and validating chronic sorrow, modifying the need for mastery, assisting in reconstructing identity, engendering hope, and facilitating the finding of meaning.[31] Such facilitation of meaning-making may include identifying spiritual understandings, cultural beliefs, and philosophy of life, and externalizing the attributions of the cause of ambiguity.[32] A process of sharing narratives within the person's family allows understanding and acceptance of different perceptions of the loss.[33]

Chronic Sorrow

Ambiguous loss may be associated with the phenomenon of chronic sorrow. Living, ongoing, irresolvable loss may produce a pervasive sadness and desolation, along with difficulties with stress management; and the chronic nature of the loss may produce "frozen grief."[34] A cycle may occur, where despair is followed by limited adaptation, and again, uncertainty and despair.[35] Outcomes may include a breakdown in coping strategies, and unresolved grief.[36] Chronic grievers may contend with "an anguishing invalidation of their central assumptions about God, the universe, their loved one and other people," and struggle to rebuild a life narrative that makes sense of their loss, their present situation, and their future.[37]

---

29. Boss, *Loss, Trauma*, 144–46.
30. Ibid., 15–17.
31. Boss et al., "Ambiguity and Uncertainty," 169–72.
32. Boss, *Loss, Trauma*, 74–83.
33. Boss, *Ambiguous Loss*, 128–32.
34. Boss et al., "Ambiguity and Uncertainty," 167.
35. Ibid., 165.
36. Ibid., 166–67.
37. Neimeyer and Currier, "Bereavement Interventions," 18.

Grieving Losses: "The Long Goodbye"

Nonfinite Loss

A closely related phenomenon is the grief associated with a nonfinite loss, a loss that may be unidentified by others as loss. This involves a "continuing presence of the loss"[38]—physical, emotional, and/or psychological—that increases over time with no clearly defined end, involves lost hopes and dreams, and engenders a significant search for meaning.[39] Characteristic of nonfinite loss are ongoing uncertainty about the future; a loss of supports; a sense of disconnection from the person's normal world; a serious challenge to one's assumptive world; a sense of powerlessness, embarrassment, and self-doubt; an absence of acknowledgment, rituals, or validation of the loss; and ongoing despair.[40] Schultz and Harris propose that support in the disenfranchised grief of such ongoing loss should include identifying what is lost and what is not lost; creating loss rituals; finding supports; validating and normalizing the grief; and facilitating meaning-making in the loss.[41] In the journey with a loved one with dementia, such nonfinite and ambiguous loss, and associated chronic sorrow, may overlap; and although often not identified as grief, may call for very specific interventions.

Empathic Failure

Disenfranchisement of grief and empathic failure in such losses may occur at one or more parts of the person's social system: at the family level, where there may be different perceptions of the loss; at the community level, where it may be overlooked; at the personal level, where some aspect of grief is disowned within the self; or at the level of self with transcendent reality, where a shattering of the assumptive world may precipitate a spiritual crisis.[42] Identifying the sphere in which empathic failure has occurred will facilitate appropriate interventions to validate the grief and to allow the mourner to reconstruct meaning through a narrative of the loss.[43] Such an intervention may draw people together in social support,

---

38. Schultz and Harris, "Nonfinite Loss," 238.
39. Ibid., 238–40.
40. Ibid., 241–42.
41. Ibid., 243–44.
42. Doka, "Disenfranchised Grief," 229.
43. Neimeyer and Jordan, "Disenfranchisement," 105–8.

facilitate emotional relief through expressing feelings, and allow people to make sense of the loss.

Grief and Dementia

Caregiver Grief

Recent dementia research and theory offer a small but growing literature relating to caregiver grief and its effects. Grief may, in fact, be the lens through which many caregivers view their caregiving responsibilities and burdens.[44] However, because of caregiving demands and because of the insidious, ambiguous, and intermittent nature of cognitive decline and loss, and the ambiguity of lucid episodes even into late dementia, there may be no awareness of grief, and help may not be sought.

Anticipatory grief, often invisible but ongoing, accompanies caregivers on the dementia journey. The meaning of this term has been broadened beyond the anticipation of a future death, and it embraces past and present losses in the person with dementia and in the relationship, including the loss of intimacy, companionship, former roles, and relationships with others. The emotional response to such losses is complicated by the person's behavioral changes, and the caregiver's diminished coping abilities due to the demands of care-giving.[45] A major early study found that anticipatory grief, experienced from diagnosis on, was not mitigated by its long-term nature and was not indicative of better post-death adjustment.[46] It was noted that as caregivers were not resolving the cyclical and sustained grief and despair on their own, there was a pressing need for adequately evaluated grief interventions that would potentially benefit persons with dementia, families, and society.[47] The study recommended support that would facilitate a review of the caregiver's life changes, address issues of role change and ambiguity, legitimize care-giver needs, and encourage access to support systems.[48] More than a decade later, a study of the impacts of anticipatory grief again identified this as a key element of caregiver burden, and again called for grief support to be provided to validate anticipatory

44. Adams et al., "Personal Losses," 313.
45. Doka, "Anticipatory Mourning," 481–86.
46. Ponder and Pomeroy, "Grief of Caregivers," 15–18.
47. Ibid., 15–16.
48. Ibid., 17–18.

grief and facilitate the expression of the full range of emotions, and thus to reduce the distress and sense of isolation in caregiving.[49]

A range of impacts of caregiver grief have been identified. Meuser and colleagues indicate that there is an interactive process, where grief contributes to caregivers' depression, stress, and burden, and vice versa; and they argue that grief should not merely be subsumed under these other effects, needing attention in its own right.[50] They identify three components of grief: heartfelt sadness and longing; worry and felt isolation; and the burden of personal caregiving sacrifice. Their research indicates significant differences between partner and adult offspring grief, and differences in grief focus across the course of the journey.[51] They argue that the intensity, pattern, and focus of the grief need to be identified for effective interventions;[52] and they propose that, to enhance coping and promote well-being, grief should be normalized through non-judgmental listening and discussion.[53]

Anticipatory grief and ambiguous loss have been found to create the biggest barrier and burden in caregiving, and long-term grief interventions are proposed, as the loss and grief do not diminish over time.[54] Research with couples following diagnosis has led to the conclusion that shared negotiation of the losses and development of coping skills early in the journey might be beneficial in coping with the ongoing losses, and that maintaining social roles was beneficial in sustaining couple identity.[55] A study of the impact of personal losses and relationship quality in dementia caregiving concludes that relational deprivation, including a decrease in intimacy and a loss of self-identity, contributes to overload and symptoms of depression.[56] In the loss of relationship and other roles, it appears that caregivers' identity may be subsumed under the caring role, and that caregivers have difficulty making sense of their own life.[57]

The differences in family members' interpretations of the loss are a considerable source of stress and grief. Bender graphically suggests that

49. Holley and Mast, "Anticipatory Grief," 388–94.
50. Meuser et al., "Assessing Grief," 175–78.
51. Ibid. See 179–86 for further explanation of research findings.
52. Ibid., 178–80.
53. Ibid., 186–87.
54. Holley and Mast, "Anticipatory Grief," 394–96.
55. Robinson et al., "Making Sense," 344–46.
56. Adams et al., "Personal Losses," 313–15.
57. O'Shaughnessy et al., "Couple Relationship," 252–54.

within the family system "many psychic injuries are caused by bits of loss and grief and anger and despair flying around."[58] Boss suggests a collaborative approach with a therapist and family members, where perceptions of the ambiguity are targeted through listening to family members' experience and facilitating meaning-making.[59] As well as facilitating cognitive processing for the reconstruction of identity, interventions with family caregivers should encourage affective processing, validating and normalizing ambivalent responses, and inviting the expression of the full range of emotions.

Grief and Persons with Dementia

There is much still to be learned about the grief of persons with dementia; but it is important to emphasize that they still experience the emotional impact of the losses. Although in later dementia they may be unable to cognitively identify the losses and may forget or become confused about what is lost—losses including their past life and lifestyle, sense of control, independence, the ability to interpret, the sense of self—there is no reason to assume that the emotions are lost.[60] Bender maintains that a person with dementia needs to accept that the losses are permanent and to relinquish past abilities and the past concept of the self; and he argues that support is needed to do this, to incorporate the losses into the life narrative, and to build a new sense of identity.[61]

While there may be debate about whether people with dementia should be told their diagnosis early, it is important to recognize the potential benefits of this knowledge. The person and partner together, while it is still possible, can work at making sense of their challenges, make plans, maintain a social identity, share in processing the losses, and support one another in the grief of the situation. Attentive listening may lead persons with dementia into exploring their grief, and they, like caregivers, will need validation and enfranchisement of their feelings. In extensive spiritual reminiscence research and work with persons with dementia, it was found that, while cognitive limitations made it difficult for some to express their grief, there was generally a freedom from inhibitions and a willingness to discuss grief and death; and spiritual reminiscence groups are proposed as

58. Bender, *Explorations*, 327.
59. Boss, *Loss, Trauma*, 88–91.
60. Killick, "Dementia, Identity," 71.
61. Bender, *Explorations*, 317–19.

an avenue for expressing grief and receiving support.[62] Further insight into the grief journey has been provided in narratives written by people during their own journey. About a decade after her diagnosis, Bryden writes:

> We need you to acknowledge who we are, to listen to our emotion and pain, and to treat us as people of value and dignity, worthy of respect.... I believe it is wrong to deny us help to deal with the whole gamut of emotions we will experience.... Grief is one of the first and most common reactions to dementia, and it is an anticipatory loss of self that is being grieved for.... We need to grieve many times, as each successive loss becomes apparent to us.[63]

Application of Bereavement Theories

This section will argue that, despite vital insights from the various bereavement theories, these theories do not fit well enough with the ongoing and ambiguous loss of the dementia journey and into bereavement. There have been some attempts at their application. Robinson and colleagues find some relevance in dual processing theory, but its application is not straightforward. They find an oscillation between acknowledging the losses and developing coping strategies and negotiating the changes together.[64] Small and colleagues note a modified "continuing-bonds" approach that proposes ongoing engagement with "the person that *was* while not denying the challenges of living with the person that *is*."[65] Such an approach conflicts, however, with the call to value, engage with, and affirm the present person rather than try to retrieve "the person behind the dementia." The model of *deconstruction* and *reconstruction,* which involves experiencing the pain of the loss and reconstructing an internal bond with a "lost" loved one, presents a somewhat similar problem where the loved one is still present and the losses are unclear and unpredictable. Although there may be major losses in the person with dementia and changes in the former relationship, the application of single pathway grief theory is not appropriate. Where the loved one's *presence* demands constant and focused care, the tasks of moving on in life and investing in other relationships are not feasible, and

---

62. MacKinlay and Trevitt, *Spiritual Reminiscence,* 184–85.
63. Bryden, *Dancing with Dementia,* 130–31. See pp. 105–13 for emotional responses to loss.
64. Robinson et al., "Making Sense," 343–44.
65. Small et al., "End-of-life Care," 381.

are certainly not appropriate in light of the person's dependence on loved ones for sustaining her/his social self. In addition, the losses increase rather than decrease during the journey, and any restorative movement towards rebuilding a new life during the exhausting journey is extremely problematic. Where the loved one is placed in a residential aged care center, often a caregiver's focus shifts to that environment, and this becomes the caregiver's world. With this change in social context and the changes in the caregiver's former identity (including now the sense of a loss of identity as primary caregiver), adjusting the sense of the self in the changed world presents a major challenge.

The extent to which these bereavement theories are applicable to caregivers' *post*-death grieving is also open to serious question. Much ambiguous and nonfinite loss may have already occurred without validation of feelings or social recognition of grief, and there may be chronic sorrow. With the possibly long and gradual change of relationship with the person and with others in the family and social network, and without time or opportunity to process the emotions or reflect on the meaning of the losses, much of the caregiver's grief may not have been processed, enfranchised, or even identified. If the person with dementia has been in a residential aged care center prior to death, the caregiver may have lost connection with any other social context, and after the loved one's death the caregiver loses this context and its support. Empathic failure may occur not only during the journey, but also during bereavement, because of assumptions in the family and social network (if that network still exists) that relief should be the caregiver's only emotion. Thus bereavement theories in general do not fit well with the ongoing and ambiguous losses throughout the journey and into bereavement.

Making Meaning: A Spiritual Task

Effective grief interventions for persons with dementia and caregivers will emerge from a multidisciplinary theoretical and empirical base; and there have been recurrent calls for further research and for interventions that prove their effectiveness in enhancing well-being over time. These calls are as yet unanswered in any significant way. One bereavement grief approach that warrants serious consideration for this journey and beyond death is that of meaning-making. This approach, with its internal and social processes for addressing grief and rebuilding personal identity, presents possibilities for interventions responsive to the grief and confusion of the journey.

A Spiritual Framework

A framework is needed, within which all insights relevant to this ongoing and complex grief may be integrated; and a key proposition of this monograph is that a spiritual framework is appropriate for the provision of effective interventions. The loss and grief—often long-term, cyclical, ambiguous, anticipatory, non-finite, unidentified, disenfranchised, and experienced in increasing isolation from a social network—are likely to be associated with the loss of identity and meaning, conflicts between beliefs and present experience, disconnectedness, and suffering. The post-death grief of caregivers, complex and unmitigated by the pre-death experience of loss, calls for support tailored to the individual needs. Identity, connectedness, and transcendence are recognized as being integral to spirituality, and the loss of meaning and connection are associated with spiritual distress.

There is increasing awareness of the spiritual dimension in well-being, an acknowledgment of meaning-making as a central element in spirituality, and an understanding that spiritual care identifies and works with what gives meaning, purpose, and connectedness. There are solid theoretical grounds for arguing that spirituality and religion may have significant impacts on grieving, through providing a system of meaning, significant coping resources in bereavement such as a belief in eternal life, and rites, rituals, and a social support network to assist in the grieving process.[66] A broad spiritual framework is appropriate for integrating significant aspects of this particular grief, and facilitating a comprehensive support system of spiritual care through the journey. Within such a framework, meaning and benefit may be found in the journey, the affective impact of the losses may be normalized and emotions expressed, the loss may be incorporated in the larger life narrative, and ongoing connection may be available to ameliorate the grief, isolation, loss of identity, and disconnectedness of the journey.

---

66. Park and Halifax, "Adjusting to Bereavement," 358–59.

Sustaining Persons, Grieving Losses
Grief Work and Spiritual Care

As we have seen, the dementia experience may bring challenges to a person's belief system, spiritual distress, and possibly despair. In the challenges to a person's assumptive world and the ambiguous losses of the journey, meaning-making might assist in identifying what is lost and what is not lost, processing the grief, exploring a person's sources of hope and purpose, and clarifying the person's spiritual and/or philosophical understandings and interpretations of the experience. While there may be an inability to make sense of this non-finite loss, meaning-making may also facilitate coping, through finding comfort in spiritual benefits including spiritual growth, compassion, and wisdom in the experience. Thus a person might discover unidentified strengths and abilities and broader purpose in the journey. If new life meaning can be found, the experience may become one of transcendence and hope rather than despair.

Listening with empathy is a substantial resource in spiritual care, facilitating significant connection, narrative, affective expression, and support. In a long-term, empathic, supportive relationship, the caregiver or the person with dementia or both together may be enabled to identify the losses, past, present, and future; and caregivers might be encouraged in grieving the losses *and* nurturing the personhood of the loved one and the self. The ongoing co-construction of a biography of the person with dementia and the integration of this journey into the person's whole life narrative would support continuity with the past, and facilitate coherence and reconstruction of the identity of both the person with dementia and the caregiver. The expression and processing of emotions might be facilitated, and ambiguity and ambivalence normalized. In the absence of the formal rituals that facilitate grieving in bereavement, during the journey a spiritual caregiver might encourage rituals that are meaningful within the person's belief system. Such rituals might acknowledge losses and grief and facilitate celebration at important milestones such as anniversaries. A spiritual caregiver could offer support at critical times such as when the person is placed in permanent care, and in the late palliative stage where verbal communication with the loved one may be difficult or impossible. Following the loved one's death, the complex grief might be further enfranchised by a spiritual caregiver who has journeyed with the grieving person.

The journey often described as "the long goodbye" calls for support throughout, and beyond the final goodbye. The grief may be disenfranchised within the person, the family, and the social context; and where it is not identified and acknowledged, grief interventions *per se* are unlikely to be sought. In any case, short-term interventions are unlikely to address grief experiences that are fluctuating, long-term, and ambiguous. Spiritual care not only facilitates the complex, interrelated cognitive-affective processes of grieving and meaning-making, but also allows the loss narrative to be integrated in the spiritual narrative of the whole of life. This long grieving may give rise to spiritual questions of identity, meaning, suffering, connection, and transcendence that may thus be addressed in spiritual terms; and an ongoing narrative incorporating this experience into a whole-of-life journey may nurture the identity and affirm the personhood of the person with dementia and the caregiver. Person-affirming relationships are recognized as crucial in sustaining persons on the journey. The persistent calls for grief interventions, support within the family system, and holistic care need to be heard; and ongoing spiritual care in the context of appropriate empathic relationship would offer consistency of connection, and support responsive to the ongoing challenges of dementia.

Within a multidisciplinary team providing services for persons with dementia and caregivers in the community, spiritual care should be as readily available as social support, domestic assistance, and nursing care. Home visits of spiritual caregivers need to be accessible throughout the journey for the individual and the family system, from diagnosis through the difficult period of placement in a residential aged care center, continuing with the person in care and the family caregiver until and beyond the loved one's death. Thus the well-being of those who travel the journey might be greatly enhanced. For those within faith traditions, ongoing building of the narrative of the journey might facilitate its coherence and alignment with a tradition's larger story, in the context of, for example, a meta-narrative of transcendence, of life triumphing over death and hope winning over despair, whereby meaning may be found in the person's suffering.

Meaning and Hope in Grief

In summary, a journey through dementia is accompanied by losses and grief—complex, ambiguous, non-finite, anticipatory, and too often disenfranchised. While research continues to explore impacts of loss on caregivers and persons with dementia, spirituality offers a framework for theory and practice in the grief journey. A spiritual approach is appropriate, then, where grief support may be offered by a spiritual caregiver who accompanies a person or a family unit on the spiritual journey through dementia, and is there for the complex grief of bereavement.

Within such a framework, pastoral care might be provided for Christians on the journey, both caregivers and persons with dementia. While the themes of suffering and hope are set in the larger Christian narrative of eschatological hope through the life, death, and resurrection of Jesus Christ,[67] theological content or platitudes must not be used by the pastoral caregiver to smother a person's suffering. Rather, pastoral care allows people to express all their emotions; to draw on their own spiritual resources; and to tell their story and make sense of it in the context of the larger narrative of faith, thus finding hope in the midst of their grief.

---

67. These themes are discussed in chapter 7.

6

Local Pastoral Practice, Perspectives, and Meanings

> *As I travel towards the dissolution of my self, my personality, my very "essence," my relationship with God needs increasing support from you, my other in the body of Christ. Don't abandon me at any stage, for the Holy Spirit connects us. It links our souls, our spirits—not our minds or brains. I need you to minister to me, to sing with me, pray with me, to be my memory for me.*
> —CHRISTINE BRYDEN AND ELIZABETH MACKINLAY, "SPIRITUAL JOURNEY."

> *So far in my pastoral ministry role here I have not had need to deal with dementia patients and will have nothing significant to contribute to your study.*
> —PASTORAL CARE COORDINATOR, EMAIL DECLINING INVITATION TO PARTICIPATE IN THE RESEARCH.

AN UNDERSTANDING OF CURRENT pastoral practices begins "on the ground," and it is from here that theological reflection leads to enhanced practice responsive to the needs of those on the dementia journey *and* grounded in the church. To this end, a small-scale qualitative study was undertaken with Christian churches of a suburban locality in Australia, to discover and reflect on current pastoral practices and their undergirding theological perspectives relating to dementia and grief. (This locality was not the one from which participants were drawn for the caregiver study.)

Focus Group Study

A focus group methodology is used for the purpose of exploring new concepts, producing concentrated amounts of data on a research topic, and interpreting its meanings.[1] Small focus groups are a means of obtaining qualitative data through focused interactive discussion concerning a question of interest to the researcher.[2] The goal of the research was to describe, and explore the meanings of, the pastoral practices of Christian churches in a geographical area. To this end, a careful and systematic content analysis of each group's data was undertaken, followed by a thematic analysis of each data set, and then an analysis across groups to consider commonalities, divergences, and gaps in practice and understanding.[3] The discussions were structured around the same set of questions in all groups, and the researcher was involved in guiding the discussion to include all topics.[4]

Research Design

Gathering Data

Again, in accordance with the Human Ethics processes of the University of Queensland, and with the specific and clearly stated agenda of exploring local practices relating to dementia and grief, prospective participants were invited to participate in focus groups, to discuss their churches' pastoral practice.[5] The groups had a reasonable level of homogeneity, as participants were all involved in pastoral care in Christian churches; and most of the participants were unknown to one another.[6] Questions were about the challenges that were confronted and steps that were currently being taken in pastoral practice, and guiding principles and theological understandings that guided the practice. The exploration included any scriptures,

1. Morgan, *Focus Groups*, 7–14.
2. Krueger and Casey, *Focus Groups*, 10–12.
3. Wilkinson, "Focus Group Research," 182–85.
4. Morgan, *Focus Groups*, 38–40.
5. See Appendix B.1
6. Morgan, *Focus Groups*, 34.

theological and pastoral writings, or other resources that were found helpful for practice relating to dementia and grief.[7] The researcher facilitated and moderated the discussions, prompting, encouraging elaboration, and following up interesting points. All participants were given opportunity to express their positions and describe their churches' practices.

While recognizing the limits of a small and not necessarily representative sample, understanding of local practice was developed by thoughtful interpretation of the data. With clear traceable steps in data collection and analysis, the description of practices was verifiable as a reflection of what participants in the process communicated. The findings are, then, indicative of the local phenomenon, and transparency in the research process allows the reader to assess transferability to other situations.[8] Although no claim is being made to a set of findings that can be generalized from this study, there are conclusions that serve as vital insights into responses to a particular situation, and illuminate some aspects of the wider context of pastoral care for the dementia journey.

Thematic and Interpretive Analyses

Thematic and interpretive analyses of focus group data were undertaken, with the underlying view that what is said provides access to what is thought, believed, and practiced.[9] The transcript-based systematic analysis sought to determine the emerging themes, divergences, and outliers; and the findings were reported using carefully chosen participant quotations to connect readers with participant experience. Strengths and gaps in practice, knowledge, and theological foundations were identified, and reporting was guided by the goal of description and understanding of practices, the researcher recognizing that she was the coordinating voice of participants. Because of a low response rate for participation in focus groups, a questionnaire was offered as a supplementary means of broadening the data. The questionnaire data were analyzed and practices described and interpreted in conjunction with focus group data. Thus a description was developed and a theoretical understanding of the local phenomenon emerged out of an interpretive process.

---

7. See Appendix B.2
8. Krueger and Casey, *Focus Groups*, 203–4.
9. Wilkinson et al., "Focus Group Research," 187–88.

The focus group format facilitated informal group discussion of participants' understandings, experiences, and practice, and explored a social question in a social context. The sampling was purposive, as the participation of all churches in the area was sought in order to gain a broad understanding of pastoral practices relating to dementia in the area. The focus group allowed a collective construction of meaning as well as insights into the pastoral contexts of the participants. The small size of groups encouraged participation by all, with the researcher inviting the elaboration of comments and follow-up of interesting points, and prompting an exploration of topics which appeared to be being avoided. This process ensured that all topics were considered and encouraged respectful interaction among the participants.

Method

Recruitment

Ministerial and church office contact details were collected from church websites and the local phone book, and contact was attempted with all local churches. Initial contact was made with twenty-two churches, by means of an email indicating the nature and purpose of the research, inviting the participation of a minister or pastoral care coordinator representing their congregation, and indicating that a follow-up phone call would be made. Where possible, this follow-up occurred within the following week, to answer any questions and personally invite participation. Follow-up contact was in many cases difficult; but where phone calls and messages were not responded to, the researcher persisted. In three cases, this personal contact was impossible because emails and repeated phone messages were not answered.

The acceptance rate for the invitation was small. One minister, two pastoral care coordinators, and three pastoral representatives nominated by their ministers/priests expressed a willingness to participate. (One representative was subsequently unable to participate, and her congregation was not represented. Three of the pastoral representatives requested that they might bring another pastoral team member.) The pastoral care coordinator of a church-affiliated Community Care service agreed to represent this local service. Thus two focus groups were set up, where five local churches and one Community Care service were represented. Seven ministers of other congregations, unwilling to participate in a focus group, agreed to contribute via an emailed questionnaire covering the same topics. One was completed and returned; two reminders were emailed to each of the other prospective respondents over a period of several weeks, without response.

Because of the small participation rate in this locality, an adjoining (and socio-economically somewhat different) area was included in the research to broaden the pool from which data were drawn. The same method of recruitment was used, and this elicited a quite similar response rate. Twenty-two churches in this locality were approached, and two focus groups were set up which accommodated those willing to participate. Four local churches were represented, with participants including one minister, two pastors to the elderly (from one church), two pastoral care coordinators, and a pastoral helper. Three denominationally employed chaplains participated, one of whom worked in the local community and two in aged care centers. Four questionnaires were accepted, two of which were completed. (Reminders about the other two did not bear fruit.)

Focus Group Process

The focus group approach facilitated participation. Groups were convened at times suitable for all prospective participants. The venues were church facilities centrally located in the local areas. Prior to each focus group meeting, information and consent forms and a summary of questions for discussion were emailed, and further phone contact enabled participants to clarify any details. Each focus group met for approximately one hour, preceded by refreshments and the collection of signed consent forms. Participants sat in an informal circle around a table. The questions for discussion were again provided to each participant. Guidelines for focus group discussion were established: respect for other participants' views, confidentiality concerning the content, and opportunity for all to participate. The researcher facilitated the meeting, which was recorded. To conclude the meeting, the facilitator briefly summarized the main points, invited comments, and expressed appreciation for the group members' participation and contributions. (The participants of one group, previously unknown to one another, conversed informally for some time following the meeting, and commented positively on the value of meeting for such a discussion.)

Thematic Analysis of Data

Immediately after each meeting, the audio-recorded group discussion was transcribed verbatim, and listened to a second time in order to capture nuances in tone, and gain insight into unfinished or ambiguous comments and pauses. The researcher sought to identify her own assumptions, biases, foreknowledge, and perceptions gained from the caregiver study, and to maintain that self-conscious stance, immersing herself in the data of one focus group at a time. Emerging themes were identified by coding key words and phrases. During the analysis the researcher sought to hear what was being said, what was being assumed in what was said, and what was not being said. Thus common themes, divergent views, and gaps or silences from unrepresented realities became evident. Significant quotes were highlighted and used within the text of the thematic analysis. Note was also taken of the interactive features of the data, a distinctive aspect of focus groups, such as participants expanding on, challenging, or ignoring the comments of others. Thus a "thick" description was developed of the phenomenon as it was represented by participants in each group. The questionnaire responses were also analyzed thematically, and pastoral practice in the represented churches was described.

Overall Interpretive Analysis

Having thematically analyzed the data provided by the groups and questionnaires, further analysis was undertaken. Using themes emerging from the process as building blocks, an interpretive analysis sought to gain a unifying perspective by asking, in the light of social scientific and pastoral/theological literature and research, "What does all this mean?"

Focus Group 1

Thematic Analysis

The participants included the pastoral care coordinators of two churches, one of whom brought an assistant. Another church was represented by two members of the pastoral care team. One church reportedly had a membership in the hundreds, one a membership of about one hundred, and the other approximately fifty.

Local Pastoral Practice, Perspectives, and Meanings

The Challenge of Not Knowing the Needs

The predominant theme was the perceived gap in communication from the family to the church concerning pastoral needs during the dementia journey. The issue was expressed by a pastoral care coordinator as, "If they [the family] do not talk to us, tell us, we're not mind readers." The barriers were seen to be the family not acknowledging the condition or keeping silent about it, a lack of trust of the church, and the family not wanting to ask for or accept help. One participant reflected: "You strike that a lot, 'oh, no, I can manage'—how do you break down that barrier?" One participant acknowledged that it might take the pastoral team some time to realize that a church member had dementia, and another stated that "there are many 'dementias'[10] out there [in her church] that we're not tapping into." It was tentatively proposed by another participant that friendships within the congregation might be a way of discovering the pastoral needs; but this was not explored. While most participants believed the onus was on family caregivers to seek support, another perspective on the issue was graphically presented by one participant whose parent had developed dementia without the family initially realizing it, "it took a long time for the penny to drop, and by the time we did realize, it was like having a tiger by the tail." This experience did not generate any discussion.

Persons with Dementia: Perceived Needs, Pastoral Response

This theme covered the receptivity of persons with dementia to spiritual practices even into late-stage dementia, and the pastoral response. One participant stated: "the spiritual dimension is the last to leave them." Six references were made to members of sacramental churches responding into advanced dementia to familiar prayers, the Eucharist, and a crucifix. One participant noted that his personal experience of a parent's dementia did not line up with the view of the person's ongoing spiritual responsiveness, referring to his deep distress, "like twisting a knife in your heart," that his parent forgot her faith. This experience was not explored for pastoral meaning.

Two participants noted the need for ongoing inclusion of people with dementia in their Christian community. Such inclusion was offered in one church through bringing people to public worship and visiting six

---

10. The participant's term for persons with dementia!

or seven at home to offer Holy Communion. The two larger churches provided monthly church services in aged care centers, and it was noted that if their church members with more advanced dementia could not attend these services, Holy Communion was taken to them in their rooms. In one church, a "friendship group" had been functioning for the past eight years. A meeting was held twice a month with an attendance of about eighty older people, including some with dementia from within the congregation and the wider community. This service provided transport, food, conversation, entertainment, and a prayer before the meal, and "has become more like a family affair."

The emotional needs of persons with dementia were touched on, briefly. It was speculated that there might be anxiety in the early stages as persons realized what they were losing, and it was proposed that a pastoral caregiver might "journey with them." None said they did. One participant noted the loneliness of people with dementia living on their own, which he had observed in the community through his "Meals on Wheels" visits: "A lot of people, it's really sad, who don't seem to have enough support, they don't get out, they want to talk and you don't have time."

One participant referred to the distress of a person with dementia in repeatedly hearing, as if for the first time, of the death of a loved one. Two participants spoke several times of the "need to keep them happy," and it was stated that a person with dementia can "enjoy the moment" into advanced dementia. One pastoral caregiver noted that her ongoing visiting in aged care centers maintained some connection with people with dementia, who continued to recognize her.

Caregivers: Perceived Needs, Pastoral Response

In response to the researcher's persistent return to the question of challenges faced by family caregivers, participants referred to a number of possible caregiver emotions including frustration, annoyance, loneliness, distress, embarrassment, fear of dangers related to the person with dementia, and grief. Two brief references were made to the distress caused by a loss of recognition of family members by persons with dementia. One participant proposed that pastoral caregivers could look after the spiritual needs, and should be able to provide information about practical and emotional supports such as local community caregiver support groups to which caregivers could be referred, for support from people "who had been through the experience." This participant commented that pastoral caregivers who had not had the experience (of a loved one with dementia) could not support caregivers emotionally.

Grief

The churches' approach to grief was briefly considered. One participant said that their church practice was to visit any bereaved families in the congregation, send a card after the death and at the first anniversary, and send families an invitation for a memorial service during the year. One person suggested that caregiver grief is a long process, before as well as following the loved one's death. There were differing views as to whether the person's death would bring relief to the family, but it was agreed that the grieving continues afterwards. One participant recalled the "emptiness" expressed by a personal friend a year after the loss of a loved one for whom the friend had cared for many years, and one suggested that even after a person has been in permanent care for a long time, death leaves a big gap.

Theological Understandings and Teaching

To the question of whether and when their church teaching or preaching addressed issues of aging, grief, and loss, there was a prolonged pause. The one response was that "pastoral care is the most important part." To the question of theological understandings or Scriptures helpful in their pastoral work for the dementia journey, reference was made to Psalm 23, the Lord's Prayer, and scriptural assurances that God will never forsake the person. One participant said she assures the person that the Holy Spirit is there.

Resources

The question of resources was discussed. One person said that inviting speakers would not be useful as people do not attend such events, and that a good library might be useful. One person had been helped by a booklet "Ministering to People with Dementia: A Pastoral Guide," but she noted that bookshops have no record of it and it might be no longer available.

There was reference to the Bible as a resource, and the booklet *Somebody Cares* (a collection of verses from Scripture) was mentioned.

Focus Group 2

Thematic Analysis

The participants included the leader of a church of several hundred, one pastoral team member who visited aged care centers representing a large church, and a church leader who was the full-time pastoral care coordinator for the local region of a large church-sponsored Community Care service.

Challenges for Caregivers

The challenges faced by caregivers constituted the main theme. The isolation of caregivers, the challenging behaviors of loved ones with dementia, and the pressures of role changes in early dementia were identified. Reference was made to the very distressing decision to place a loved one with dementia in permanent care, with examples of a husband struggling with a sense of breaking his marriage vows, and a wife with a sense of failure in being unable to continue caring for her husband.

The ongoing losses were seen as a significant challenge for family caregivers. References were made to the impacts of changes in the loved one's personality: for example, where a daughter struggled to love her changed parent, and where a grand-daughter felt that her grandmother had "gone already." A participant shared her personal experience of deep distress in not being recognized by a parent in later stage dementia, and sadness in the parent's being unrecognizable as the same person. One person stated that the loss of the person as she had been was a source of long-term multi-layered caregiver grief.

Challenges for Churches

A second theme was the challenge of continuing to include persons with dementia and caregivers in the congregation. In one congregation, strong individual friendships, a pastoral care network, and an awareness of individuals' needs within the groups to which they belonged were seen as important in maintaining connection. This participant acknowledged that they "could still slip through the cracks. The biggest challenge for us . . . is how to ensure they stay embraced as part of the community, a very big issue." He commented that their church as yet had "no specific care regime" for those with dementia.

The inability of caregivers to continue with activities in the congregation was noted. There was agreement that families usually do not inform their church of their needs in caregiving, and it was suggested that this is possibly because in the early stages they may go into "coping mode" rather than having time to think about their challenges or about asking for help, and later it may seem too late.

Pastoral Responses to Caregivers

There was discussion about means of pastorally supporting caregivers experiencing the "multi-layers of grief." One participant suggested that for caregivers, it was a struggle and a journey toward acceptance, and she used both listening and "talking them through." She said she often offered follow-up grief support after the loved one's death, where again "talking them through" the grief helped them to cope and understand that they had already been grieving. One participant suggested that listening during the journey was the key, "exploring with them what is actually going on at a deeper level."

Pastoral Responses to Persons with Dementia

One participant spoke of visiting persons with dementia and sharing the Eucharist in their home, listening and building relationship with them, and at times advocating on their behalf with community nursing staff. She gave pastoral opportunities for exploring a person's thoughts and fears about the future.

Two represented churches were involved in aged care center worship services. Ministers and lay people from one church conducted weekly services in two aged care centers, where residents with dementia were included. The participant reflected that some who conducted these services attempted to gear the service to connect with residents with dementia, while others took the position that where "the body" was gathered, God was somehow present to them. This church had denominational chaplains who visited centers to support residents pastorally, including those with dementia. A second participant belonged to a pastoral team that visited one aged care center weekly to offer the Eucharist and pray with residents, including those with dementia. Their priest conducted Mass in the center monthly, and several people with dementia attended.

In the palliative stage, ministry to persons with dementia and their families was said to be the same as for anyone else, with prayer, Holy Communion and, in some cases, anointing being offered the dying person. It was suggested that these rituals brought a sense of connection and peace for the person. The question was raised by one participant as to whether this approach "is enough, when it comes to this very particular experience of dying."

Theological Understandings and Teaching

One participant spoke of a theology of grace rather than works that needed to be integrated into life and thinking *before* the challenges of dementia, giving an understanding of God working on our behalf and holding us when we cannot hold onto God. In this church, a sermon approximately once a year focused on issues such as loss and grief, aging, and transitions. This participant referred to the presence of the Holy Spirit in the painful journey, scriptures such as Romans 8 ("nothing can separate us from the love of God" and "Christ is interceding for you") and John 10 ("no one can snatch them from the Father's hand"), and prayers and lament psalms giving expression to the struggles.

Pastoral Resources

Views varied on resources that might assist in pastoral care for the dementia journey. Ambivalence about educational resources was expressed by one participant who concluded that education "never goes astray" but that the pastoral role for the dementia journey simply required caring people. Resources in one congregation included input by chaplains, and services of remembrance from time to time for bereaved people. One suggested that it would be helpful to have some simply written material to offer caregivers early in the journey, to help to normalize their experience. Two participants found familiar prayers, Psalm 23, and old, familiar hymns helpful resources for ministering to those in later stage dementia, and the "Footprints" poem was mentioned as a resource reminding people of God's continuing presence with them.

Focus Group 3

Thematic Analysis

The participants included two "Pastors to the elderly" from a church with a membership of approximately five thousand, the pastoral care coordinator of a church of approximately two hundred members, and chaplains representing two Christian denominations in the local area, one serving in a church-related community service organization and the other in a denominationally-based aged care center. The latter was invited to participate after a leader from a local church with approximately seven hundred members indicated—as a reason for his non-participation in the research—that their denomination provided "quality care for persons with dementia" through the denominational aged care center adjoining their church, where pastoral care was provided by a chaplain.

Caregivers' Challenges

There was a focus on challenges facing family caregivers. Cognitive and physical deterioration, aggression, and changes in persons with dementia were identified as impacting on their caregivers. Points raised were a sense of shame in families, the emotionally draining responsibility of caring, and the isolation of caregivers because of the care demands. As one said, "the one who's looking after her mum at home . . . 95% of her life is cut off . . . there's not a whole lot of life unless someone comes in to give her a break . . . so much isolation."

Note was taken of the challenges faced by caregivers when loved ones with dementia were placed in aged care centers. There was a reference to feelings of guilt, and one person suggested that it was difficult initially for a caregiver to step back from over-involvement in the person's care, and then to cope physically with constantly visiting the loved one. An absence of pastoral support from the church to caregivers after the entry of their loved one into an aged care center was noted by the chaplain, as causing hurt and a loss of contact with their home church. Concern was expressed for caregivers, in that while they might develop connection with the aged care center worship community, there was no longer a church community with which they felt connected when their loved ones died.

The comment was made that grief was experienced in the ongoing loss of persons as they had previously been: "Personality changes, body decays, seems like they're dying before your eyes." Reference was also made to grief at the time of death, where people with dementia might not recognize family members at their bedside, and being frightened, might tell them to leave. Incidents were related that compounded grief: when a family enquired of a clergyman concerning their very ill loved one's funeral, they were told, "don't bother me with that now, wait till he's dead"; and when a clergyman visited a dying person in hospital, he "asked all the family to leave so that he could do his job," and then left with barely a word to the family. It was suggested that caregivers often experience, as part of their grief following the loved one's death, relief and associated feelings of guilt and shame about the relief.

Challenges Faced by Persons with Dementia

There were few references to the experience of persons with dementia. Aggression and the failure to recognize the family were noted, but only in relation to the impacts on the caregiver. The need for a person with dementia to come to an acceptance of being in permanent care was referred to, but again in relation to easing caregivers' burden. One participant raised the question of what constitutes quality of life for persons with dementia. He suggested that for some there might be a sense of fulfillment, while for others, a sense of despair. There was no discussion of what might contribute to the difference.

Pastoral Response to Caregivers' Needs

It was proposed that, especially in the early stages, family members needed someone to talk to, to process feelings of guilt and shame. One participant cited a family caregiver who would not have disclosed her situation because of shame and embarrassment, if the pastoral caregiver had not initiated conversation; and she suggested that it was crucial to allow caregivers to talk and debrief about their challenges. She noted: "I would visit the caregiver . . . I could only listen to her; . . . she said, 'It's just good to be able to say it without any condemnation.' That's all I did."

Pastoral care for caregivers included facilitating reminiscence about the loved one's earlier life, acknowledging the devastating impacts of dementia, and encouraging family preparation for the funeral as the person with dementia approached death. One participant said he offered reassurance and affirmation of caregivers' sacrificial care when they experienced relief and accompanying feelings of guilt following a loved one's death.

In both churches, support for caregivers and members with early dementia was provided through the inclusion of both partners in the usual social activities and friendship in church groups, with some practical support where caregivers were given respite by leaving their partners with friends at church social group meetings. In some cases attendance at church was possible for both partners, but it was noted that that might not continue to be possible in later dementia.

Pastoral Response to Persons with Dementia

Worship services were provided in four aged care centers by one church's pastoral team, and weekly services were held in the aged care center where the participant chaplain was based. The importance was noted of reading scriptures to people who had valued them, because of their responsiveness to them even in the later stages of dementia. Familiar scripture verses, hymns, and the Lord's Prayer were seen as meaningful, though it was acknowledged that "it's all individual" and each person needs to be accepted "where they are at the moment." One person saw the building of trust, a sense of safety in relationship, and touch as important in pastorally caring for persons with dementia. One participant noted the importance of individual reminiscence and storytelling. Another spoke of one distressed person with early onset dementia who, with no religious background, grasped the truth that "Jesus loves me," and found peace with God.

The aged care center chaplain expressed concern about church members being neglected by their church after moving into permanent care, though their church was close to the center. She said the effects of this were that residents were distressed about being ignored, and the staff observed an absence of care from the church. The participant quoted a church member who was a resident of the center: "I'm just at a loss . . . I'm just not sure how a woman of my size can be invisible." The participant added, "She's passionate about her friends [from their church] who are there who do have dementia and they have no visitors."

Potential barriers to offering appropriate pastoral care were noted. These included the feeling of "intruding in their world" in secure dementia care units, aggression shown by some, and the danger of stereotyping people with dementia. A participant spoke of the challenge of dealing sensitively with the replacement of a person with dementia on the church board, but noted this in relation to supporting this person's caregiving partner. One participant suggested that when a person with dementia was dying, the family might want assurance about her eternal future, but it was not possible to discuss this with the dying person in the same way as with someone without cognitive impairment.

Education and Resources

The topics of loss and dying were addressed in workshops in one "Older Members" group. It was noted that although younger family members were invited, they did not attend. One person suggested that pastoral care teams should know what secular community resources are available for the dementia journey, in order to guide family caregivers toward these.

Focus Group 4

Thematic Analysis

The participants included the coordinator and one member of the pastoral care team of a church of approximately two hundred, the minister of a church of approximately eighty people, and a minister serving as full-time chaplain in two large church-affiliated aged care centers. (One prospective participant, unable to attend, later provided data via a questionnaire.)

Caregiver Challenges and Pastoral Responses

Caregivers' challenges constituted the main theme. These were seen to include grief, loss of connection with the loved one, emotional turmoil, family tensions because of different means and levels of coping, and the fear of "going the same way" as a parent with dementia. An absence of connection and a sense that relationship is a "one-way street" were seen as emotionally draining for families visiting loved ones in aged care center dementia units, and a possible cause of families discontinuing visits. One participant reflected on family members' grief: "Many times I've heard a family member say "that's not the mum or dad I grew up with" . . . so they are grieving . . . they've already lost their parent." This participant explained that he spent time allowing caregivers to process the grief, encouraging them to see the loss as a "loss of relationship" with the person. There was agreement that families continue to experience grief following the person's death, and that this grief is possibly more difficult because of guilt feelings about the relief that the caring burden has been lifted.

The consensus was that support for caregivers was the principal pastoral responsibility. Two participants saw listening as the most important pastoral response to the grief, family tension, fear, and other emotional challenges: "Primarily listening . . . listening becomes a really significant issue, because families need to talk, and need to have somebody who listens to their issues, their struggles, how they've been impacted by it."

One person saw keeping in touch and "being there" for caregivers as important elements of pastoral care; and she mentioned the church's "prayer chain" where family caregivers could phone for prayer support, and a daytime home group where a person could be listened to, cared for, and prayed for. Connection was also maintained through mailing the weekly church newsletter to caregivers unable to attend services; and a mid-week service had recently been introduced in the hope of including caregivers and their loved ones with dementia. In the two aged care centers where the chaplain served, the chaplain expressed sympathy following deaths by sending a card and another on the first anniversary, and families were invited to a memorial service during the year.

Needs of Persons with Dementia

Some needs of persons with dementia were acknowledged, though one person suggested that they are in "their own little world" and it is the caregivers who most need support. One participant said that in early dementia persons were likely to be aware that they were forgetting, while still believing that they were "very normal." It was suggested that this might be a frightening and frustrating experience, causing them to cling to their independence and resent its loss, prompting anger towards their loved ones and feelings of embarrassment and hopelessness. It was proposed that later there would be a sense of isolation, an absence of connection, and grief: "they may mourn their own loss . . . inwardly grieve because there are so many things they have lost." One participant drew attention to the impact on persons with dementia of other people's responses and stress in the environment.

Pastoral Response to Persons with Dementia

Identifying one's own reactions, showing respect, and avoiding being judgmental were seen as important in relating to the person. One participant suggested that "commiserations" should not be offered to persons struggling with the emotions engendered by their losses, that the experience should not be seen "as a negative." His practice was to encourage people to give thanks to God for what they still had rather than focusing on what they had lost. Another participant agreed that encouragement rather than pity should be offered.

One participant stated that it was important to connect with persons with dementia and "enter their world, . . . try to travel the journey with her, because it's real to her," and to continue seeking to connect even when it might be difficult to know whether visiting was of any comfort or significance to the person. Connecting persons with their past practice of prayer and with their past life through remembering and talking was seen as important. A participant spoke of showing honor and respect and treating the person "as you normally would," which would be helpful for the family as well as having a spiritual impact on the person. Another participant noted that respect was expressed by not imposing one's own values or preferences—such as particular music—on persons who could no longer express their own preferences.

Pastoral ministry in aged care centers varied. The aged care center chaplain said that connection was maintained with some congregation members who became residents, but it "depends on the church" as to whether members were visited after entering the centers. A pastoral team from one of the represented churches conducted worship services in four aged care centers, and teams from four churches conducted services in the centers where the chaplain ministered. The chaplain said he encouraged such ongoing connection, as "that's their identity."

Theological Foundations

Some theological insights were offered. One participant said he worked from the basis that all are spiritual beings created in the image of God, and that persons with dementia remained spiritual beings, still connected with God. He reflected: "every time you meet with someone, there's something spiritual going on, and how you respond to the person will impact spiritually." He expressed the belief that where there had been Christian faith, God continued to walk with a person with dementia and there was no difference between this person and anyone else in the church, as "all are one in Christ."

Resources and Education

Attitudes to resources for the dementia journey varied. One participant found the Psalms to be a rich resource because of their familiarity to many people and their pattern of moving from despair to praise; and familiar prayers and hymns were found to offer comfort and meaning. This participant had used "a couple of resources which reflect a Kubler-Ross grief process," and would encourage people to access more qualified help if he deemed it necessary. Another said that he had an *ad hoc* approach and had not looked for resources because when faced with a situation it was too late to begin researching. In reference to resources for grieving families, a participant referred to the support and resources offered by the Alzheimer's Association; however, no participant knew of any caregiver who had accessed support from this source. The Alzheimer's Association had been invited to address a "Ladies' Group" in one congregation, and there had been a positive response to the provision of information and literature. One church offered an annual six-week course, *Living Victoriously*, designed for people in their later years and addressing issues of aging, grief, and death.

Questionnaire

Data and Meanings

Three questionnaires were returned, providing data from churches of approximately sixty, one hundred and twenty, and one hundred and sixty members. While approximately one third of members in the first congregation were over sixty-five, there reportedly had been no persons with dementia or family caregivers in the congregation during the previous five years; in the second church, there were reportedly three persons with dementia and three caregivers among the thirty-three members over sixty-five, and in the third congregation, of forty members over sixty-five years, there were ten caregivers and ten people with dementia.

The pastor supplied data for the smallest congregation. Members led monthly worship services in aged care centers, with a format of songs, a short talk, and a cup of tea; and there were the joys of mutual encouragement, friendship, and seeing God working in people's hearts. Consistent ministry, if possible provided by the family and the church, was seen to be the key to meeting the emotional and spiritual needs of people with dementia. The perceived needs of caregivers included coping strategies, support, and strengthening. The pastor's personal experience of having had a parent and a sibling with dementia contributed to an attitude of patience and sympathy. Though there were no persons with dementia in the congregation, if there were they would continue to be part of "the body," needing help and support. If questions concerning the meaning of this experience were raised, the response would be an explanation of "the fall and its consequences." If a congregation member were dying, whole-congregation support would be given, with follow-up bereavement support by the pastor and deacons. In sermons annually, the theme of grief was addressed from a biblical perspective with a message of hope, comfort, empathy, and peace from God's presence. Pastoral care in grief situations involved presence, listening, encouragement, prayer, and practical support. It was suggested that biblical and relevant materials would be helpful in caring for persons with dementia and caregivers.

The response from the second church was provided by the pastoral care coordinator. The congregation conducted a monthly "normal format" service in one aged care center, with non-mobile residents having access to the televised service in their rooms. Contact had reportedly been maintained with members with dementia in aged care centers, through "visits by available people." Persons with dementia were seen as "members with special needs," needing company and spiritual reminders of what they had known in the past. Caregivers' perceived needs were for respite and encouragement, and they reportedly received visits and prayer. If questions were raised concerning faith in the dementia journey, people would be offered answers from the Bible and, if needed, referral to Christian professionals. Pastoral care for congregational members experiencing grief was provided by the pastoral care coordinator, with "full-on care" at death, including the funeral. To the question concerning teaching or preaching on themes relating to grief, he gave "death" as the answer. Though two couples from the congregation were on the dementia journey, there was no indication of resources accessed. The respondent suggested that printed information and a listing of Christian professionals might be helpful.

The respondent for the third church was the pastoral care coordinator. Monthly church services were held in aged care centers, using a shortened version of the Anglican Holy Communion order of service. It was noted that "we must meet the residents where they are at," and though it was a challenge to engage residents for the whole service, there was joy in providing opportunities for them to participate. Friends, ministers, and laypeople from the pastoral care team visited members with dementia who had entered aged care centers. Their primary emotional and spiritual needs were listed as "to be cared for, to be understood, and to be loved." If persons with dementia expressed concerns about their journey, the respondent would seek to bring peace and comfort, and would remind them of God's care for them. The needs of caregivers were seen to include respite care, support from family and friends, and understanding of their situation by their family, friends, and clergy. Prayerful and practical support was offered, with an innovative roster system whereby caregivers could receive respite while other parishioners cared for their loved ones. This provision was gratefully accepted by some, while others "have been stoic and not responded well." Pastoral support was given by the clergy at the time of death, with continuing support for bereaved people through a follow-up system involving the clergy, lay people, and possibly someone with experience in the dementia area. The respondent had been helped by the *Spark of Life* dementia program, which had made a significant difference in the aged care center where her family member had lived. There had been no preaching or teaching on grief or dementia in the congregation during the previous ten years, and the respondent suggested that a workshop and a discussion group on dementia-related issues would be helpful.

Overall Interpretive Analysis

Research Data

The level of participation in this research project is noteworthy. The invitation to participate was extended to the priest/minister/leader of each church in the local area, with the option of delegation to the pastoral care coordinator. Where the focus group invitation was not accepted, a questionnaire was offered. Of the forty-five churches contacted, nine were represented in focus groups and three via questionnaires. The participation rate for clergy was small. In spite of the researcher's persistence and willingness to accommodate ministers' schedules in meeting times, and notwithstanding the offer of the questionnaire as an alternative means of participation, only two ministers representing local churches and two pastors (from one church) participated in the focus groups, and one pastor via the questionnaire. Four locally based aged care/community chaplains represented three different Christian denominations.

The actual data then relate to a small number of congregations whose representatives took the time to reflect and respond concerning their pastoral practice and theological perspectives. The contributions of participants, all involved in pastoral practice and some having accompanied family members and personal friends on the dementia journey, are particularly important, representing possibly the most intentional local pastoral ministry to people on the journey. The limited discussion time of about one hour may mean that identified gaps in the data are not necessarily indicative of actual gaps in practice. However, as participants had time to consider the topics beforehand, and as groups were small enough to allow participation by all, it might be expected that the most salient information was provided. Likewise, those who completed the questionnaire had time to reflect in making their response.

Bringing together the data from focus groups and questionnaire responses, an interpretive analysis is undertaken. Meaning is sought through the analysis of common themes, divergences, and gaps in practice and theological understanding across data sets. Several questions are addressed, including: the participants' perceptions of pastoral needs of persons with dementia and their caregivers; the means of responding to the needs and the meanings of these pastoral responses; the gaps in practice and their meanings; the attitudes toward resources and any gaps between currently accessed and available resources, and between available and desired resources; and the principles and theological concepts that undergird and guide practice. The practice, meanings, values, and gaps then provide a local starting-point for enhancing the practice of pastoral care for the dementia journey.

Commonalities, Divergences, and Meanings

Diversity

Different perspectives and priorities for pastoral ministry in the dementia journey were articulated in different groups. Much was verbalized in one group about pastoral care through the provision of sacraments to persons with dementia, while in two groups the priority was clearly pastoral care for caregivers, especially through listening. There was some reticence to articulate the needs of the journey, which might suggest that an underlying awareness from personal or pastoral experience had not necessarily been applied in pastoral practice. There was divergence in the pastoral responses to those on the journey. It was proposed in two groups and one questionnaire that caregivers needing emotional care should be referred on to others, to secular community support groups where others on the journey could provide support, and to Christian professional counselors; responses in two other groups indicated a sense of responsibility to "be there" for those on the journey. Interestingly, though deep compassion and sensitivity were communicated in many of the comments and activities of participants, there was only one reference to an *empathic* pastoral response (from the questionnaire respondent whose congregation included nobody on the dementia journey), and only one reference to persons with dementia needing to be loved. The differences in perceptions and focus across participants and churches indicate considerable diversity in understandings of what constitutes pastoral care, and in pastoral practices for the dementia journey.

Challenges for Caregivers, and Pastoral Responses

Perceptions of the challenges faced by caregivers and the pastoral responses to caregivers varied among groups, but with some commonality. Increasing care demands, changes in roles, isolation of caregivers, ongoing changes in the loved one with dementia, and guilt feelings were issues gradually elicited in discussions. While in three groups listening was seen as important in enabling caregivers to debrief and work through issues, listening was not mentioned at all in the other group. In three groups there were references to friendship as a means of being aware of needs as they arose and of maintaining contact within congregations, and two references to "journeying with them." There were two references to intercessory prayer support. Intentional practical support was provided for caregivers in two participating churches, through a respite program, and through inclusion of persons with dementia in a church social club while caregivers had respite. Participants in two groups suggested that pastoral teams might offer practical help by providing information about government services and respite.

The ongoing grief of caregivers was identified in all groups, with references to loss of relationship and progressive changes and losses in the loved one. The pain of not being recognized by a loved one with dementia was noted by three participants, drawing on personal and pastoral experience; and the distress of finding a person with dementia unrecognizable as the same person was mentioned twice. Two participants referred to pastoral care in the grief of the journey through intentional listening to explore the layers of grief, and one of these "talked people through" the grief. The references to listening and the one reference to allowing reminiscence during the complex grief of the journey are noteworthy; otherwise, there was apparently no practice that was responsive to caregivers' complex grief. In particular, attention is drawn to participants' reflections on caregivers' grief at their loved ones' entry to aged care centers, and to one participant's acknowledgment of the need for pastoral care more specific to caregivers' grief around the death of a loved one with dementia. These insights offer ground for building such a practice.

The pastoral care for caregivers when their loved one was dying and afterwards reportedly did not differ from that given to others facing bereavement, with one exception: one participant said she addressed the complex bereavement grief by explaining the concept that they had already grieved. There were references in two groups to a sense of guilt associated with the relief of bereaved caregivers; in two groups, to the large gap left after long-term caring; and in two groups, to the possible disconnection from the church community because of the journey of caring. The deep grief of not being recognized or wanted by the dying loved one was noted once, as was caregivers' possible concern about the loved one's eternal future and the inability to communicate about such spiritual issues. Varying experiences of the post-death grief of caregivers were noted, including absence of emotion, possible relief, guilt, and a long-term sense of emptiness. However, these levels of awareness of ongoing and post-death grief apparently did not translate into ongoing pastoral practice that *intentionally* addressed these issues. The appropriateness of "talking a grieving person through" post-death grief with an explanation that the grieving has been done was not questioned.

Pastoral Care for Persons with Dementia

Some commonality emerged in the theme of spiritual practices for people with dementia. With two exceptions, the represented churches provided worship services and the sacrament of Holy Communion for residents (including some with dementia) in aged care centers. There was consensus across groups that those in late stage dementia were still responsive to the sacraments, familiar prayers, and hymns. There were three references to attempts to tailor services to the needs of persons with dementia, with short simple sermons related to familiar experiences and in one case, with an interactive conversational style. Two participants referred to taking Holy Communion to residents in their rooms when they were no longer able to attend services. In one case services were televised to residents' rooms, but there was no indication of how or whether residents with dementia accessed them. One participant referred to transport to worship services for some people with dementia, and two referred to sharing Holy Communion with people with dementia in their homes. There was one reference to the importance of an awareness of the person's past spiritual practices for facilitating spiritual connection.

The relational needs of people with dementia received a little attention. One church's regular "friendship group" meetings provided social connections with others in the church and the wider community. One participant spoke of engaging with a person in conversation about his music interests, and two spoke of effective pastoral care arising out of relationship, where a sense of safety and trust were built with the person. Two participants referred to the value of connecting a person with her past through allowing her to reminisce. There was one reference to ongoing friendship in spite of communication difficulties, one to building pastoral relationships through offering Holy Communion to people at home, and one to the importance of giving honor and respect to persons with dementia. No insights were offered about how relationship was established and sustained, or how connection and communication were facilitated with people with diminished, fragmentary, or lost verbal language.

There was little common ground in the provision of emotional support for persons with dementia—and apparently little support. Some participants referred to emotional challenges such as anxiety and fear of the future, and the possibility that they might grieve their losses. One reference was made to pastoral opportunities to discuss fears of the future, and one to continuing to give love, comfort, and understanding through the journey; otherwise there was silence about emotional support for persons with dementia in their loss, grief, and fear at any stage, including at the time of diagnosis, relocation, or the palliative stage. The practices mentioned, while touching people's lives in some ways and providing a local base line for local pastoral practice, raise questions concerning what is understood by "pastoral care" and about underlying values and attitudes relating to the personhood, identity, relationality, and spirituality of persons with dementia.

Invisibility

A significant theme in three focus groups was the difficulty of identifying or maintaining contact with those in the congregation facing the challenges of dementia. While in two groups it was seen as the responsibility of church members to identify the needs and maintain connection, in a third group the problem was seen as caregivers' silence and failure to trust the church and ask for help. A personal insight was offered into the caregiver experience early in the journey—the experience of turmoil in the realization of a loved one's dementia; and the suggestion was made that caregivers may go into "coping mode" rather than asking for help. These examples, along with the speculations about caregiver silence, invited but did not produce further exploration of reasons for caregivers' reluctance to seek support, or for their possible disappearance from congregations, or for congregational friends' and pastoral caregivers' unawareness of the needs.

Admission of church members with dementia to aged care centers raised pastoral issues where there was little indication of responsive practice. There were two references to the challenges faced by caregivers at the time of their loved one's relocation, and one to supporting caregivers at this time. There was no reference to intentional pastoral support for a person with dementia at the time of relocation. Although there was involvement by most represented churches in worship services in aged care centers, there were only two indications that participating churches intentionally continued the pastoral connection with members who had entered permanent care. This gap in practice was highlighted by a center chaplain concerned about churches' pastoral neglect of their members in aged care centers and family caregivers who visited loved ones there, in some cases daily. While suggesting that the church was "their identity," another chaplain said that churches varied in whether connection was maintained.

Blessings in Caring

There were indications of pastoral care being a source of blessing. One participant, in sharing her "best story," spoke with enthusiasm of the peace of one person with dementia in responding to the gospel for the first time. One person commented on the mutuality of blessing, and those who shared in worship services in aged care centers conveyed the sense of joy in this ministry. On the other hand, it was noted that people might tend to stop visiting and maintaining relationship with people with dementia because this can be draining. Apart from two references to entering their world, and two to "going with the flow," there appeared to be a general perception of pastoral care being done *to* persons with dementia, mainly through worship services and the sacrament of Holy Communion. Mutuality in pastoral relationships and enrichment through such relationships with persons with dementia were not considered.

Resources and Education

It is informative to consider the resources for the dementia journey used currently by these pastoral practitioners. Scriptures, and in particular Psalm 23, were the main resource referred to in all groups, the value of their familiarity being noted. One participant had found a respected secular dementia training program helpful. Another had used a booklet, now unavailable, on pastoral care and dementia, and a chaplain had used some Kubler-Ross material; neither was a recent publication. There were no indications that any participant had tried to access any recent resources.

Theological Foundations for Practice

There were some commonalities and some individual perspectives concerning theological underpinnings for practice. In all groups the theological concept of God's ongoing comfort through the presence of the Holy Spirit with persons with dementia was expressed. In three groups, scriptures expressing the concept that God would not abandon the person were seen as important. The commonalities ended there. One minister referred to an overarching theology of grace, of "God holding us," which needed to be integrated into life *before* the challenges of dementia and aging. There was one reference to the belief that God is present in a special way in the gathered community, one to there being a spiritual dimension in all interactions with people, and another to Jesus' very direct, honest, and compassionate model of ministry, of being present with the person needing healing. There was one reference to the promises of Romans 8 and Christ's intercession for us. One person's belief that "we are all one in Christ" meant that there was no distinguishing pastoral response for this journey. A questionnaire respondent believed that persons with dementia continued to belong in "the body" (though there had been none in his congregation in five years), and he alone referred to hope. These practices and theological foundations are the context within which gaps in practice and theological understanding are discussed, and meanings sought.

Gaps and Their Meanings

Participation in Research

The level of response and the attitudes conveyed concerning the research project warrant attention. 80 percent of churches contacted were unrepresented in focus groups, and less than a quarter were represented at all. Reasons given for non-participation are noteworthy. Two ministers of churches with over one hundred members did not participate because, they said, there were no caregivers or people with dementia in their congregations and therefore they had nothing to offer. The leader of a church of 500 members stated strongly that his ministry team members were much too busy to contribute to "such research" as this. A "pastor to the elderly," representing a church with a membership reportedly in the thousands, said she was too busy to attend a focus group. After agreeing to receive a questionnaire, she later emailed saying that she "did look through the questionnaire you sent me and decided that the work that I am doing has no relevance to the work you are committed to." The pastoral care coordinator of a church with a reported membership of approximately three thousand replied by email to the invitation, saying: "So far in my pastoral ministry role here *I have not had need to deal with dementia patients* and will have nothing significant to contribute to your study" (emphasis added). The pastoral care coordinator of another church with a membership in the thousands, who was to be going away "later" and was too busy to complete a questionnaire, wrote "as a Pastoral team we commit to helping our church family through any disease or challenge that arises as best we can." The leader of a congregation of over a hundred members forwarded his pastoral care coordinator's response, which read:

> My thoughts on these matters could be written on a postage stamp. My very limited experience extends to [two named couples where one partner had dementia and the other was the caregiver, in the congregation]. One hour in a group discussing this topic is not my ideal.

Such attitudes and levels of participation in the research suggest that this pastoral area is not widely perceived by local ministers and pastoral care coordinators to have even a moderate level of priority or relevance.

Reported Incidence of Dementia in Congregations

The small percentages (and the absence) of persons with dementia and caregivers reportedly in congregations raise significant questions. With the general "graying" of church congregations, it might be expected that the incidence of dementia and caregiving in local congregations is at least comparable to that within the general population. In Australia, at about the time the research was conducted, it was estimated that about 9 percent of people over sixty-five had dementia, the prevalence increasing to about 30 percent of people over eighty-five. Over 50 percent of persons with mild dementia and over 34 percent of those with severe dementia were living in the community.[11]

In light of these statistics, questions must be raised when ministers of churches of a hundred or more members reportedly across all generations say that they do not have, and have not had in recent years, caregivers or persons with dementia in their congregations, and when the reported numbers of people with dementia and caregivers in almost all participating churches represent very small percentages of reported congregational numbers. Are people on the dementia journey present in congregations

---

11. Australian Institute of Health and Welfare, *Dementia*, 12–21.

but "invisible?" If so, why are they, why are family caregivers not seeking pastoral support for themselves and their loved ones, and how are they coping? If they are no longer in congregations, why are they not, and how are they coping? If it is suggested that well over half of the residents in aged care centers have dementia, and therefore many people with dementia are no longer in congregations, further questions are raised. Who maintains pastoral relationships with people who are no longer able to participate in congregational life because of such relocation, and with family caregivers who remain in the community and continue to care for their loved ones living apart in residential aged care centers? Who supports disconnected and isolated caregiver members emotionally and spiritually when they face the complex grief and loneliness of the journey and bereavement?

There was apparently a general unawareness of people on the dementia journey disappearing from congregations. Where the reason given for non-participation in the research was a lack of any members on the dementia journey presently or recently, no explanation or excuse was given for the absence. Research participants, with two exceptions, did not reflect on the possibility of having lost contact with members facing dementia challenges. One chaplain expressed concern about the emotional and spiritual impacts that such loss of connection might have on caregivers who were already isolated, and on people with dementia who could no longer participate in the activities of the church community.

The major gaps in the available local data raise broader questions. Is the response to this research limited because in local churches there is little awareness of the issues of the aging population, or little or no concern for them? Do ministers not see their leadership as encompassing theological values and pastoral practice related to aging, suffering, and grief? What attention is given to other vulnerable and grieving members of these congregations? What spiritual nurture is provided to the aging and suffering, if questions of loss, grief, and care for the vulnerable and grieving are not addressed in the churches' preaching and teaching? And what theological understandings and values underlie these gaps in the data concerning the local practice of pastoral care in general, and during the dementia journey in particular?

Local Pastoral Practice, Perspectives, and Meanings

Gaps between Experience and Pastoral Practice

An exploration of participants' references to their personal experience of the dementia journey proved interesting. Though nine of the participants had first-hand experience of a loved one with dementia (partner, parent, sibling, or friend), it was not generally apparent (with exceptions) that their *personal experiences* had illuminated their pastoral practice, nor were their own experiences readily incorporated into the focus group discussions of pastoral needs or practice. For example, no connection was made between the "failure" of families to ask for help, and a participant's personal experience of an uncontrollable situation of suddenly realizing a parent had dementia. There was no discussion of the disparity between the concept of "spiritual awareness" into late dementia and a participant's personal pain of a loved one forgetting God. Such experiences as these, and one participant's deep distress and sadness in being unrecognized by a parent and being unable to recognize the parent as the same person, might have opened windows to discussion of both responsive practice and relevant theology.

Pastoral *experiences* did not appear necessarily to expand pastoral practice. Pastoral encounters were narrated that acknowledged spousal distress about placement of loved ones in residential aged care centers, but only one participant referred to supporting a family caregiver at this time. There was no other reference to pastoral practice addressing caregivers' distress, grief, and guilt feelings prior to, at the time of, or in the months and years following the loved one's residential placement. References were made to pastoral encounters indicating difficulty in loving a changed person, and a continuing sense of emptiness a year after a loved one's death, but these insights apparently had not influenced current pastoral practice, nor were they explored in the groups for pastoral relevance.

There was some theoretical and experiential knowledge of the long-term nature of the journey, but this did not generally appear to translate into consistent, long-term pastoral support. There were few indications of support for caregivers in their ongoing and changing emotional challenges. There were no references to intentional, regular visiting of isolated caregivers who could no longer connect with their congregation in worship or activities. There was no reflection about the impacts of a long journey on caregivers, and no indication of whether pastoral friendships with caregivers endured throughout the journey. Any dilemma presented by grieving the losses while focusing on the positives was not discussed. There were few indications of validating feelings or offering empathy, and none to any rituals acknowledging grief or milestones during the journey. Questions were not raised about *how* the church might facilitate communication with caregivers and encourage openness about the needs, *why* caregivers might experience embarrassment and shame, *how* these feelings might be ameliorated, and *why* there might be a lack of trust or expectancy of receiving support from their church.

Gaps in Practice

No pastoral practice responsive to the *spiritual* challenges of the journey was elaborated. There was no reflection on *spiritual questions* arising from issues raised: for example, a loved one's forgetfulness of God; or a caregiver's possible spiritual pain in a sense of disconnection from the local congregation; or the support of a loved one's identity or of a caregiver's own identity; or God's presence or absence in an experience which might challenge their whole belief system. One participant referred to the church prayer chain which caregivers could access for support, and two to prayerful support; there was no other reference to ongoing prayerful support, or prayerful presence, or intercession in the midst of the challenges.

A pastoral role within family systems was not elaborated. While there were references to friction within families and one acknowledgment that family tensions affect the person with dementia, there was no discussion of the importance of the family system for the quality of life of persons with dementia. While there were two references to aggression from persons with dementia toward caregivers, there was only one reference to pastoral conversations that included both persons together, even early in the journey with couples who together belonged in the congregation. While it was acknowledged that relocation of persons with dementia into aged care centers was very difficult, and especially so for caregiver-partners, there was no reference to pastoral support for caregivers or couples together or families in that often traumatic life change.

The silence about the ongoing journey of both caregivers and residents after entry into a center highlights the concerns raised by a center chaplain. Where do people find a place to belong in the church when they live in aged care centers, especially if their center does not provide pastoral support or worship services? Who accompanies caregivers and persons with dementia on this part of their spiritual journey, and supports them at the end of life? And where and how do caregivers receive pastoral support and reconnect with their former church congregation following the death of their loved one with dementia, if they have been isolated from that congregation while supporting their loved one in a center, possibly for years?

Gaps in Knowledge and Application

There were gaps in dementia-related theoretical knowledge and its pastoral application. While one person stated that spiritual needs and awareness continued into late-stage dementia, there appeared to be an assumption here that spiritual needs equated to sacramental, religious practices. One reference was made to the sensate awareness of persons with advanced dementia, but no application of this knowledge was apparent in making relational connections, or in making spiritual connection with one whose religious heritage might not have focused on sacraments and icons. Music was referred to in relation to familiar hymns, and there were two references to touch, but there was no other reference to the senses or exposure to nature in connecting with people or connecting them with their past or with God. It was acknowledged by one person that persons with dementia need love, and there were two references to listening and presence. Nothing was said in any group about ways of connecting or communicating with or relating to a person who had lost cognitive processing and verbal skills, or about means of connecting spiritually, or sacred presence, or intercessory prayer, with persons with dementia.

There were few references to pastoral relationships with people with dementia. While listening was acknowledged to be a significant tool for supporting caregivers, this was mentioned only once in relation to people with dementia who might be trying to make sense of the journey. It did not appear that there was intentional emotional support for persons in early dementia, though loneliness and the possibility of anxiety and fear about memory loss were noted across all groups. Though reference was made to the recurring grief for a person with dementia in repeatedly forgetting and rediscovering that family members had died, this was not analyzed in relation to pastoral practice. The validity and implications of the theory expressed in two groups that persons with dementia needed to be "kept happy" were not questioned in relation to their possible grief about their losses. Indeed, it was suggested that they should receive encouragement rather than pity, and that the pastoral caregiver should not "go there" (into grief) or commiserate with them. The approach of avoiding their grief by encouraging a focus on what had not been lost presents the dilemma of sustaining the present person *and* validating grief, but this was not discussed. No participant referred to questions of faith, spiritual pain, or the impact of a possible sense of loss of identity, or fear of loss of connection with God or other people. Mutually enriching relationships with persons with dementia were not mentioned.

Gaps in Resources and Training

Approaches to accessing and offering resources for this pastoral ministry require attention. One participant suggested the desirability of printed material with personal stories of the journey, which might normalize caregivers' own experience. Apparently none of published personal stories had been accessed in any groups, and no such resources were suggested as potentially valuable for persons with dementia early in the journey. Secular caregiver support groups were suggested as a resource that might be accessed for emotional support, but there was no acknowledgment of this being a *spiritual* journey where spiritual challenges might call for discussion and support in such groups. The possibility was not considered of spiritually sensitive support groups for persons with dementia, or for couples or family units negotiating the challenges of dementia. There was no reference to recent literature relevant to this area of ministry coming out of pastoral studies or from social scientific sources, or to recent literature relating to grief in general or the particular grief challenges of dementia. While there was a suggestion that a church library would be a good resource, there was no indication that any library or bookshop had been accessed for this area of ministry.

Attitudes to training for such pastoral ministry must be noted. No training of pastoral care teams about dementia or grief or listening was mentioned, and little interest was expressed in the possible provision of resources for such training. One participant's comment about educational resources invites further reflection:

> When I first read that, I thought we ought to tell our teams what dementia is about and what it entails, but really, as pastoral carers, our job is to walk beside, and just to share God's love, we're never alone . . . yes, education never goes astray, but I think that faithful people who generally want to care for persons with dementia or

carers, it's just that simple ... if you've got that education, great, but I don't think you need it in the end.

In light of the increasing incidence of dementia, the level of community awareness and media attention, the constantly increasing body of dementia research and literature, and books on pastoral care and dementia, such a view raises questions. Considering the dearth of resources accessed by these ministers and pastoral caregivers who are obviously committed to their pastoral task, and the absence of pastoral education about dementia, one might ask: does this expressed view reflect the prevailing attitude among pastoral caregivers, and if so, is it appropriate? *Are* pastorally caring people "walking beside"? *Is* caring for people on this journey "just that simple"?

Gaps between Practice and Theology

The spiritual and emotional challenges and pain of the journey raise theological questions for those on the journey, those giving pastoral care, and the church as a whole. The participant's pain of the "twisting knife" caused by his parent's forgetting God raises the question of a theology that might ground and sustain both the persons with dementia and their caregivers through the whole journey. Reference was made in another group to a theology of God's faithfulness, God's remembering and carrying the person though she might forget God; and this son's pain cried out for such a perspective. In relation to this gap between theology and experience, the reflection of one minister/participant is worth noting again, that theology needs to be integrated into life *before* such challenges come. While this minister's church provided preaching annually on such topics as grief, lament, suffering, and aging, the responses of other participants would suggest a gap generally in their churches' preaching, teaching, and application of theological concepts relevant to these areas of life.

While a theology of God's faithful, ongoing presence in the journey was articulated, the available data relating to local practices raise the question of how or whether this is lived out through the faithful, ongoing presence of Christ's followers throughout the journey. The theological concept of a God who does not abandon may be a consolation in the challenges, but it may be difficult for some people to reconcile this concept with a sense of being abandoned by God's people on a journey into loss, isolation, forgottenness, and forgetfulness. While these pastoral caregivers were involved in ministry and religious practices to persons with dementia, the description of pastoral practices did not indicate, in significant measure, sensitivity to the possible spiritual and emotional pain of the journey, or application of theological concepts relating to grief, identity, belonging and connection, or hope. (There was one reference to hope in a questionnaire, and none in focus groups.) There appeared to have been no discussion of these pastoral and theological issues within local pastoral care teams or churches.

There was no articulation in the groups of a theology of the church as "the body" where the members need one another, love one another, and support and give honor to the more vulnerable. The question of why people might feel shame and embarrassment and might not seek pastoral support indicates possible theological gaps relating to the personhood and place of the person with dementia in Christian congregations, the practice of pastoral care, and the role of Christians in developing a supportive loving community. The theological statement of one aged care center resident distressed by her church's perceived neglect of their elderly members in the center, especially those with dementia, was quoted by a participant: "they're building an empire by dismembering the body . . . that is the body of Christ that is being dismembered." The statement invites attention.

Directions

The findings of this local research project raise the question: "Where to from here?" The participants were all involved in leadership and/or pastoral care to the older cohort in their congregations. Compassionate and passionate commitment to their pastoral task was clearly evident, and joy in their ministry was real. Their practice and their churches' practices of pastoral care in the dementia journey have been described. In one group, one participant reflected on the possible need for a care regime specifically for those on the dementia journey. In another group one person, reflecting on the churches' limited pastoral resources, suggested that churches generally "do not do it well." He noted the need for intentionality in this ministry, and raised the possibility of training and support provided by a "broker" to churches interested in this ministry. He added that training would be useless unless a church had "a focus on loving your neighbor, loving someone with dementia."

The insights of these participants and the practices of care they describe are glimmers of light, beams and shafts of light in a darkening landscape for those on the dementia journey in this local community. In response to the insights gleaned through this qualitative research, the question of a comprehensive pastoral practice throughout the journey must be considered. What is an appropriate pastoral response to the journey? Whose responsibility is this? And what theological concepts might undergird and inform the practice? Engagement in theological reflection takes account of the findings of this study and the challenges and needs identified in the caregiver study, in light of knowledge from cultural sources; and such reflection will lead to an enhanced practice responsive to the pastoral needs of this journey. This is the task at hand.

7

Theological Foundations for Care

An individual life can flourish only in the context of a flourishing community, a community that seeks to honor, value, and include in its common life all of its members, particularly those who are most vulnerable and therefore in need of hospitality and friendship from others.
—SUSAN MCFADDEN AND JOHN MCFADDEN, *AGING TOGETHER*

Loneliness is the suffering in suffering. To experience oneself as abandoned, forgotten, neglected, and forsaken smothers one's sense of belonging and identity in the wider spiritual community.
—PHIL ZYLLA, *ROOTS OF SORROW*

AN APPROPRIATE MODEL OF pastoral care for the dementia journey takes account of relevant research from cultural sources and also the lived experience of people on the journey and current pastoral practices of care. It is as we reflect theologically on these insights through the lens of scriptural principles that an informed Christian pastoral response emerges.

The caregiver study participants have experienced ongoing burden and loss, at times agonizing, in their caregiving journey. During a year's journey, five caregivers face certain and uncertain future losses, including the feared loss of recognition by the loved one and the dreaded placement of their loved one in permanent care; and two endure existential loneliness in the absence of their partner. All partners indicate that something of their own as well as their loved one's former identity has been lost. In their losses and grief, there are few indications of anyone journeying with them. Although they endorse the value of talking, there is generally little opportunity to share their story or that of their loved one with anyone other than friends struggling with similar issues, where time and opportunity are limited. There is little other indication of empathy in their challenges. In fact, based on their experience, doubt is expressed by several that anyone else *will* understand; and the contrast between the responses to their experience and the warm support for people with physical illness reinforces this doubt. Emotions are suppressed, expressed in private, or shelved for fear that if expressed they may overwhelm. Grief is disenfranchised, generally unidentified by caregivers' families and in their networks. It is a long and lonely grieving. It has been difficult to make sense of the journey, though most find purpose in their caregiving.

These caregivers have been sustained in their caring by spiritual values and practices, faith, and prayer. However, for those connected with churches there is disappointment with their churches in this spiritual journey. For four, corporate worship is inaccessible, frustrating, or discouraging. There is a desire for, but an absence of, corporate or pastoral prayer support. There is no ongoing pastoral care for them or their loved ones. There are few indications of congregational members providing practical help or supportive friendship. In this context there is empathic failure, and these caregivers have a sense of disconnection between their personal spiritual journey and the Christian community.

From the churches of the research locality, there are varied responses to the dementia journey and grief. It appears from the level of non-participation that the enhancement of this pastoral ministry has a low priority for the majority of church leaders in that locality. There are few indications that church leaders or pastoral representatives theologically address questions of aging and grief with their congregations; and there are few indications of planning or equipping for an informed and comprehensive response to the emotional and spiritual challenges that aging and suffering may present to their members. Apparent indifference to issues pertinent to an aging population, and gaps in both the articulation of relevant theological principles and the expression of pastoral care for the dementia journey raise serious questions. Is there a convincing rationale for establishing a model of care to be applied in the church community, or would the effort be better spent in engaging with the health care sector to promote the value, and to advocate the inclusion, of spiritual care among the community services provided for the dementia journey? Are there distinctively Christian concepts and practices that offer more solid ground than the shifting sands of community standards, priorities, and mores? In a nutshell, why bother with Christian pastoral care for this journey?

Theological Foundations

Pastoral care, if it is to be genuinely Christian, must ground itself in Scripture, theology, and the resources of the church, including its fellowship, rather than reflecting a prevailing worldview. It is generally acknowledged that the health and peace of individuals cannot be separated from the health and peace of the communities to which they belong. In light of this, for some time there has been concern that approaches to Christian pastoral care do not take the building of healthy congregations seriously enough, for, while the personal approach to pastoral care is not wrong, the congregational dimension is vital.[1] While we acknowledge that the personal struggles of life are significant, a privatized pastoral approach that aims merely to help people adjust to the prevailing conditions is inadequate. Rather, pastoral care calls for an eschatological faith which lives out "a fellowship of reconciliation—with God, within the church as the body of Christ, and within society."[2] Pastoral work bears witness to the coming reign of God at each of these levels when it facilitates reconciliation, healing, and hope, and as it creates and restores enduring relationships of love and respect.[3] The church, composed of those in whom Christ is being formed, reflects the essence of the gospel in responding to *real* human need in *real* situations and offering *real* care as part of a common humanity, rather than in being, as Lyall puts it, "a 'holy huddle,' furtively isolating itself from the world."[4]

While a model of Christian pastoral care must take account of the prevailing attitudes and practices of the church, its foundation lies first of all in what the church is called to be, rather than in its current expressions. If practices are to be enhanced and the body of Christ built up, it will be as we articulate and build on theological foundations. The pastoral challenge of the dementia journey is part of a larger challenge, the challenge of how a Christian community might sustain persons, foster meaning, address suffering, encourage hope, and invite people to live their lives within the larger

1. Lyon, "Congregational Studies," 261–62.
2. Purves, *Pastoral Theology*, 148.
3. Ibid., 147–49.
4. Lyall, *Integrity*, 95.

Christian Community

So what are Christian communities called to be and to offer pastorally? The apostle Paul uses the metaphor of the human body (1 Cor 12:12–27) to depict "a community that is a supernaturally created unity with diversity" where each member belongs, baptized into and connected within the body by the Spirit and given the Spirit to drink.[5] Reflecting the unity and diversity of the Godhead, this metaphor indicates that members are interdependent, individual, and indispensable, called to value all members, to care for one another, and to give special honor to the more vulnerable, "so that there should be no division in the body, but that its parts should have equal concern for each other. If one part suffers, every part suffers with it; if one part is honored, every part rejoices with it" (1 Cor 12:25–26). The understanding of all members being integral and bound together is reinforced in Paul's letter to the Romans, where he explains that while all members do not have the same function, in Christ we form one body where "each member belongs to all the others" (Rom 12: 5). Paul follows his body metaphor to the Corinthians with "the most excellent way," elaborating the quality of the love that is life-blood of the body, a quality of love that "always protects, always trusts, always hopes, always perseveres" (see 1 Cor 13:1–8).

Called to Care

The church's true identity, then, is revealed in discovering what it means to be a community committed to loving God and one another, and living out of the love flowing from the "community of love" that is the Trinity.[6] Such a task carries both great privilege and weighty responsibility. The New Testament scholar Victor Furnish, arguing that "the one enduring reality, apart from which humanity cannot flourish, is love (*agape*)," points out that if we, the beneficiaries of this love, fail to be its agents—especially to the weak in faith—we sin against Christ Jesus.[7] The Parable of the Sheep and

---

5. Witherington, *Conflict and Community*, 261.
6. Swinton, *Dementia*, 158–60.
7. Furnish, *New Testament Theology*, 97.

Goats underlines both the sobering consequences of withholding love, and the high privilege of living in and living out of the flow of this love. Those who have ignored need, who have neglected the vulnerable, and who have withheld *agape* love are judged, for "whatever you did not do for one of the least of these, you did not do for me" (Matt 26:45); while those who have shared food and clothing with people in need and have offered hospitality to the stranger have had the privilege of serving Christ himself.[8]

The positive aspect of the parable highlights the need for communities where empathic hospitality is given to strangers—including persons with dementia and their caregivers who may become "strangers" to one another—and where people are invited to move from suffering to hope and from being strangers to belonging.[9] Such hospitality, where one makes oneself and one's space available to be with others in their suffering or confusion, offers a stark contrast in a world where there are attitudes of self-interest and non-availability, where one's existence is seen as a possession to be withheld for fear of its being dissipated.[10] In a culture that is uncomfortable with the experience and the expression of suffering, others' or one's own, empathic engagement with those who suffer may be counter-intuitive.

Love and Friendship

Agape love, hospitality, and interdependent relationships are then essential qualities of Christian community, the body of Christ. In light of the isolating experiences of those in our caregiver study, and the isolation and loss of friendship spoken of by many traveling the dementia road, we must address the question of how and on what basis these qualities are to be expressed in Christian communities—in practice, rather than merely in theology. In their instructive book that discusses dementia, friendship, and community, Susan and John McFadden argue that in a culture that views friendship in terms of social transaction, congregations are to be "schools for subversive friendship, subversive because they do not follow the script of the prevailing culture."[11] Our attention is drawn to the divine community, the Trinity, with its "mutual indwelling in love," as our model and empowerment for

---

8. See Matt 25:31–46.
9. Swinton, *Dementia*, 268–71.
10. Pembroke, *Working Relationships*, 25–28.
11. McFadden and McFadden, *Aging Together*, 147. See pp. 132–48 for an elaboration of a congregational role.

such communal life.[12] Indeed, Jesus himself, on the last night of his earthly life, spells out to his close disciples the quality and source of such mutual love and friendship.

> "As the Father has loved me, so I have loved you. Now remain in my love.... Love each other as I have loved you. Greater love has no one than this, that one lay down his life for his friends. You are my friends if you do what I command.... This is my command: Love each other." (John 15: 9, 12–14, 17)

Jesus' model of sacrificial friendship demonstrates commitment, inclusiveness, and self-giving love. It is as we abide in the love of the Father and the Son that we have a divine quality (and an inexhaustible quantity) of love to offer one another and the "stranger"; and in the sharing of this love there is the possibility of making God real in the world. As human beings we *need* to belong in community; and as we create places of hospitality and belonging and relationship, as we live in love and suffer in solidarity with and for our neighbor, we live out the image of the God who invites humanity into friendship-relationship with God through Jesus Christ.

Abiding in the self-giving love of the Father and the Son provides solid ground for the qualities of genuineness, participation, acceptance, and empathy in pastoral relationships, where we seek to step into the world of the other with understanding and compassion; and in their expression, these qualities are a reflection of the *agape* love, presence, compassion, and acceptance revealed in the incarnation.[13] Such a quality of friendship calls for reciprocity rather than a hierarchy in caring,[14] for it is obvious that as we make space in our lives to step into a person's world, we stand on the same level rather than above the person. Pembroke points out that such self-giving love requires work, time, energy, and grace, as we empty ourselves of our own concerns and our self-focus to be truly and actively present with the other.[15] This may be costly; yet it is with such God-given love and mutuality in care that all are sustained in relationship and in community. This responsibility and privilege challenges the church to continue to explore ways in which its community life can more effectively share this quality of

---

12. Pembroke, *Renewing Practice*, 43.
13. Lyall, *Integrity*, 95–101.
14. MacKinlay, "Friends and Neighbours," 72.
15. Pembroke, *Renewing Practice*, 45–47.

love with those on the dementia road who may be becoming "strangers" to themselves and to those around them.[16]

Suffering and Community

Loneliness

In the suffering that dementia brings, there is often an experience of deep loneliness in the stories shared by persons with dementia and caregivers. Such loneliness is echoed in the stories of several in our caregiver study located in different church contexts, where suffering is largely a solitary affair without expression, acknowledgment, or hope. In the churches represented (and unrepresented) in the research, it appears that there may be gaps in addressing suffering and engendering hope. A Christian leader's offering of platitudes for the caregiver in deep grief, another leader's reference to being positive and not "going there" into grief with a person with dementia, a pastoral care coordinator's suggestion that empathy and emotional support are the province of secular support groups, and the absence of teaching or preaching on grief suggest a culture that denies or ignores suffering, and implicitly judges those who cry out in lament or anger. As Pattison states, if theology is to be taken seriously, it must take all dimensions of embodied human existence, including the emotions, very seriously; we cannot ignore aspects of existence that are important to human beings themselves, or hide dimensions of life that would be destructive if not acknowledged[17]—for if we ignore suffering, we leave suffering people alone and lonely. Where such a culture exists, we must work to change it.

The impacts of such loneliness are significant. Zylla aptly describes loneliness as "the suffering in suffering," where persons feel themselves cut off, unseen, unacknowledged, not understood.[18] As he expresses it: "all suffering is difficult to bear; suffering that is borne alone is excruciating and nearly impossible to express."[19] He spells out the possible reasons for this experience of suffering and abandonment: physical pain can be so agonizing that it cannot be expressed, or understood by others; psychological anguish may emerge from the loss of former meanings and convictions

---

16. Swinton, *Dementia*, 258–60.
17. Pattison, *Practical Theology*, 189–90.
18. Zylla, *Roots of Sorrow*, 72–76.
19. Ibid., 72.

that sustained us; social belonging, companionship, and connection may be disrupted or shattered; and a sense of spiritual abandonment, being cut off from God, may thrust us into "the dark night of the soul."[20] As Zylla explains, the anguish of suffering includes the isolation of being unable to express the inexpressible; and the experience of abandonment is accompanied by yearnings to be seen, to be understood, and to belong in a community of belonging.[21] In seeking to nurture healthy Christian communities, we must ask how such anguish can be acknowledged and how these yearnings are to be addressed, not only in the isolating journey through dementia but in all the afflictions of life.

Lament Expressed

In giving voice to suffering and reducing its loneliness, the Hebrew Scriptures provide a rich source for reflection. The Psalms acknowledge *all* aspects of life, including anger, disorientation, and conflict between belief and experience. Some analyses of the lament psalms emphasize the movement from lament to praise; but it is important not to gloss over the validity of lament that acknowledges "the complexities, ambiguities and the untidiness that characterize much of human existence."[22] Indeed, the psalms of lament "do not simply reflect our experience; they are meant to *form* our experience of despair," as they lead us into honest expression of our emotions, name the silence in our suffering, and bring us into communion with God and one another.[23]

The reading of these psalms may give voice then to feelings of doubt, fear, or despair that otherwise remain unexpressed, in the suffering associated with dementia and many other challenges. Often cited as particularly relevant to the experience of dementia, Psalm 88 testifies to "the integrity with which Israel approached experiences that ran counter to its more 'comfortable' theological utterances,"[24] in permitting the expression of theological ambiguities of suffering, and in allowing a person's deepest needs to be satisfied by lament. This personal lament witnesses to the possibility of

---

20. Ibid., 58–66.
21. Ibid., 120–26.
22. Villanueva, "*Un*"*certainty*, 255.
23. Hauerwas, *Naming the Silences*, 82, italics in original.
24. Mandolfo, *God in the Dock*, 193.

unrelieved suffering for a Christian,[25] where all that might ease the suffering is the psalmist's persistent crying out to God in the darkness. In the psalmist's descent toward death, the source of despair is the sense of rejection and isolation from God and human contact:

> I am set apart with the dead,
> like the slain who lie in the grave,
> whom you remember no more,
> who are cut off from your care.
> You have put me in the lowest pit, in the darkest depths.
> Your wrath lies heavily upon me; you have overwhelmed me with all your waves.
> You have taken from me my closest friends and have made me repulsive to them. I am confined and cannot escape; my eyes are dim with grief.
> Why, O LORD, do you reject me and hide your face from me?
> From my youth I have been afflicted and close to death; I have suffered your terrors and am in despair.
> Your wrath has swept over me; your terrors have destroyed me.
> All day long they surround me like a flood; they have completely engulfed me.
> You have taken my companions and loved ones from me; the darkness is my closest friend. (Ps 88:5–9, 13–18)

Addressing God in the confusion of suffering, then, is modeled in the Hebrew Scriptures. Where there is incongruence between the core claims of covenantal faith and lived experience, and where there is deep need, Israel chooses to tell the whole truth.[26] The psalmists experience and express the ambiguity of God's presence and absence, the ambivalence of hope in the God who saves and despair when God's face is hidden, the tension between faith in the God of covenant love and the present experience of the God who has abandoned, and the silence of God in response to the persistent question of *why* in undeserved suffering. For Job, too, undeserved sufferings prompt the question *why*, to which God responds not with condemnation but with a different question; the question of *who* broadens Job's perspective and shows him himself under the providential care of the God of the universe.[27] In fact, the point is worth underlining that it is Job's friends

---

25. Kidner, *Psalms*, 319.
26. Brueggemann, *Theology*, 378–81.
27. Hopson and Rice, "Book of 'Job'," 95–97.

who are judged not merely for their false comfort, their lack of empathy, and their unwillingness to allow Job authentic expression in his suffering, but also for not speaking truthfully about *God*.[28] We as the body of Christ need such integrity, if we are to support one another in calling out to God amid life's challenges and suffering.

Lament Heard

Pastoral work, then, has an important role in encouraging people to cry out in their anguish to the God who has already drawn near to them in redeeming love; and opportunity should be given for authentic expression of people's deep distress. However, lament is seldom part of the church's worship. If suffering is not acknowledged in congregational gatherings, if praise is paramount, it is easy to infer that happiness is the normal state of the Christian and the church, and to deny oneself and others the honest expression of emotions. How isolating this can be for persons yearning to be understood in the depths of their despair! In contrast, the psalmists' almost simultaneous acknowledgments of God's presence and absence, God's love-and-faithfulness and God's abandonment indicate the paradoxes that confront faith. Where there is confusion and perhaps guilt in concurrently experiencing two opposing emotions, the ambivalence of affect articulated in some of the lament psalms (for example, Pss 13; 22; 31; 42) may normalize the experience and bring comfort.

At times, the depth of suffering may be inexpressible. Where words are no longer accessible to a person with dementia, the feelings are no less present; and we would do well to reflect on the experience of inexpressible suffering described by Zylla, as it might relate to the experience of a person who has lost the verbal ability to express the anguish:

> The mute stage of suffering is severed from the normal rhythms of life, and here, in the void of wordlessness, the suffering person turns in on himself or herself. It is an extreme and agonizing gap that leaves one unable to speak, unable to share, unable to express the depths of anguish of the soul . . . the capacity to say what is happening is cut off and the afflicted feel themselves to be godforsaken.[29]

---

28. Ibid., 89–93.
29. Zylla, *Roots of Sorrow*, 86.

It is not, of course, only a person experiencing the losses of dementia firsthand who suffers the inexpressible. Caregivers too may experience the inexpressible anguish of the soul. The wife of a prominent church pastor, Robert Davis, shared about her own experience in the epilogue of her husband's autobiographic writing concerning his dementia journey. She says:

> Sometimes in weakness and despair I want to give voice to that primal scream starting way down in the hidden recesses of the lungs—down where the ever-present knot that lives in my stomach resides—let it whirl through that vortex that's sucking my life and being into that black hole of never-ending pain, emptiness, and loneliness—just give it voice as it rises and explodes through the top of my head—Noooooooooooo! Anything, God, but this![30]

Lament Validated

In the intense sense of isolation in suffering that persons with dementia and caregivers may experience, the corporate reading of lament psalms offers the opportunity to give voice to this experience. The public use of psalms such as Psalm 88 invites the expression of anger, gives voice to the cry of despair, and allows the enfranchisement of grief for past, present, and future loss. Perhaps if such psalms were included in corporate worship, if emotions were validated and grief was shared, suffering might be ameliorated before the depths of isolation and despair were reached. Where the present situation is in conflict with a Christian's assumptive world, surely the unanswered *why* of undeserved suffering expressed in the Scriptures permits and legitimizes the questions of those who seek and cannot find meaning in their grief.

Furthermore, in a culture that often avoids or minimizes suffering, the liturgical use of Psalms might encourage understanding and compassion. Jacobson uses cognitive dissonance theory to explain the potential value in the life of the community of the liturgical use of psalms of lament.[31] He explains that where people voice words expressing emotions other than those they are currently experiencing, the disorientation that results from cognitive dissonance might foster *deeper awareness* in those not suffering, and so change their attitudes and behaviors. (He also points out the value

---

30. Davis, *Journey into Alzheimer's*, 140.
31. Jacobson, "Burning Our Lamps," 91–93.

of psalms of reorientation, for those who are suffering.)³² Such heightened awareness and changes in attitudes toward suffering may in turn foster healthy, empathic communities, where sufferers experience a sense of belonging and kinship rather than alienation and aloneness.

Responding to Suffering

Compassion

God's response to suffering should be foundational for our response. As God has moved and continues to move toward humanity in the incarnation and the cross, and in our continuing story, so we are called into the suffering of others. Jesus' ministry expressed the compassion of God in tangible, embodied ways. As Zylla puts it:

> He was not indifferent to the spiritual, physical, emotional, and social suffering of those with whom he came in contact. He was alarmed by it, motivated to help, and always responded to these situations with a gut response of concern, help, and mercy.³³

In Jesus' ministry and in the stories he told, this "gut level" compassion is powerfully evident. The Parable of the Good Samaritan (Luke 10:30–37) sharply contrasts the indifference of not seeing and of avoiding, with the compassion of coming near and entering into the suffering of the stranger in an outworking of sacrificial love—and let us not overlook the conclusion of the story, where Jesus asks which of the three was the neighbor of the suffering person: "The expert in the law replied, 'The one who had mercy on him.' Jesus told him, 'Go and do likewise'" (Luke 10:36–37).

The stories Jesus told echo and reinforce his own life and ministry, which in its entirety exemplifies his drawing near to the individual with the physical, relational, and spiritual touch of deep compassion, and his response of compassion to those who draw near and reach out to him. He sets aside his own plans, as in the meeting with the woman with "an issue of blood" (Mark 5:25–34); he touches the leper; he disregards the stigmas imposed by his culture in accepting the outcast and the needy; he sets aside his own need for rest and retreat, responding in compassion to the crowd who follow him, seeing them in their need as "sheep without a shepherd"

---

32. Ibid., 95–97.
33. Zylla, *Roots of Sorrow*, 100.

(Matt 9:36). And in his own extremity when moving toward his death, on approaching Jerusalem he weeps over the city (Luke 19:41) and reveals the depth of his yearning and compassion for those who will kill him:

> Oh Jerusalem, you who kill the prophets and stone those sent to you, . . . how often I have longed to gather your children together, as a hen gathers her chicks under her wing, but you were not willing. (Matt 23:37)

Suffering and the Cross

In the context of the new covenant, questions of suffering and grief are brought into clear focus through the cross of Jesus Christ. While there are opposing theological perspectives as to whether God suffers or remains immutable and beyond the experience of suffering, a trinitarian understanding of God's relationality sees the passion and death of Jesus as producing the "unique pain associated with the rupture in the relationships in the Godhead."[34] Moltmann reflects: "The Son suffers dying, the Father suffers the death of the Son. The grief of the Father here is just as important as the death of the Son."[35] The uniquely divine aspect of Jesus' suffering does not detract from the comfort that human sufferers can find in his human suffering;[36] indeed, through the cross, "God has entered into solidarity with the abandonment and dereliction of the human plight."[37] In this we are provided with a basis for trusting that those to whom we offer pastoral care are comforted by a God who understands their grief, who participates in their suffering, and who comes near to them by the Spirit in empathic love. The intrusion of suffering into the Christian's life can then be accepted as a sign of the fellowship of Jesus' suffering, with grief-work a subjective participation in the cross; while to avoid suffering, others' or one's own, is antithetical to both grief-work and the cross.[38] To offer pastoral care, then, in the light of the cross and God's *agape* love is to invite the expression and the transformation of human suffering and vulnerability.[39]

---

34. Pembroke, *Renewing Practice*, 105.
35. Moltmann, *Crucified God*, 243.
36. Pembroke, *Renewing Practice*, 105.
37. Purves, *Pastoral Theology*, 219.
38. Latini, "Grief-Work," 93–94.
39. Lyall, *Integrity*, 101.

Solidarity

The communal aspect of suffering cannot be overlooked, for as the apostle Paul says, "If one part suffers, every part suffers with it" (1 Cor 12:26a). Hauerwas argues that there is something wrong if Christians try to make sense of suffering *apart from* their belonging in a specific community, a people called through conversion into the fellowship of the Trinity; and if our Christian convictions are to mean anything in suffering, it will be as they help us see our lives, our narratives, located in God's narrative and community.[40] Hauerwas reflects: "historically speaking, Christians have not had a 'solution' to the problem of evil; rather, they have had a *community of care* that has made it possible for them to absorb the destructive terror of evil that constantly threatens to destroy all human relations."[41]

Comfort

If we are, then, a community of care, a community grounded in the love of God, why is it that people may experience a deep loneliness in suffering, in the body of Christ? Phil Zylla sees our tendency to avoid suffering and to withhold compassion as having its roots in a "natural" response of indifference, where we fail to see the need, we fail to acknowledge the situation, and we fail to act in love—and he suggests that this indifference is more common among Christians than we like to admit.[42] The findings of the studies herein offer some support for this assessment. The attitude commonly indicated in both studies is that understanding and empathy cannot be expected of those who have not experienced dementia first-hand; and the gaps in the pastoral response of leaders and congregations would suggest a failure to see the need, acknowledge the situation, and act in love. As Zylla points out, "compassion is costly and demands our full participation in the situation of suffering itself"; and we prefer to avoid what might cause us pain.[43] He articulates a theology of a restorative, limitless compassion rooted in the covenant love and compassion and actions of God, "the Lord, the Lord, the compassionate and gracious God, slow to anger, abounding in

---

40. Hauerwas, *Naming the Silences*, 52–54. Italics added.
41. Ibid., 53.
42. Zylla, *Roots of Sorrow*, 91–98.
43. Ibid., 94. For reference to flawed theology propping up indifference, see pp. 96–98.

love and faithfulness" (Exod 34:6); and he argues that our entering deeply into the suffering of others, owning the context of suffering as our own, and committing ourselves to addressing its root causes not only depicts God's compassionate nature, but also expresses the central mission of the people of God.[44]

How then is this compassion to be translated into an experiential, "on the ground" comfort that sustains those who suffer in Christian communities, and reaches beyond to touch and embrace those suffering alone beyond our communities? A pastoral understanding of comfort must take account of the person and work of Jesus Christ in a Christian's life.[45] Second Corinthians 1:3–5 makes this clear:

> Praise be to the God and Father of our Lord Jesus Christ, the Father of all compassion and the God of all comfort, who comforts us in all our troubles, so that we can comfort those in any trouble with the comfort we ourselves have received from God. For just as the sufferings of Christ flow over into our lives, so also through Christ our comfort overflows.

It is in receiving Christ's comfort that we become mediators of that comfort in God's ministry to the body and the world, proclaiming in *deed* that God does not abandon those who suffer but brings consolation and empowerment in suffering. If we ignore our own suffering, we set ourselves apart from the comfort and healing of Christ. It is as we experience for ourselves the comfort of the Father of compassion that we will not run from or be indifferent to the sufferings of others, but will seek to enter their world with the overflowing comfort of Christ.

Hope

As grief is articulated and expressed in the context of the gospel, and as Christ's compassion is shared and experienced in the body, hope emerges. The cross testifies to God's becoming vulnerable *for* us and thus allows us to express our brokenness and grief; the resurrection, "death defeated, speaks of hope in the midst of despair, of life transcending death, of God *with us*."[46] In this hope, God has included our history and our present expe-

---

44. Ibid., 99–110.
45. Purves, *Pastoral Theology*, 194–97.
46. Lyall, *Integrity*, 102.

riences. For Christians, then, hope is rooted in God and brought to full expression in the person and work of Jesus Christ, whose reign of love is both present and a foretaste of the ultimate victory of that reign over suffering.[47] There is a tension between the "present and not yet" aspects of this ultimate victory, where present sufferings may be difficult to reconcile with faith in the triumph of Christ over evil. This is addressed by the apostle Paul, who contends, however, that the Christian can take the future victory into account, persevering in hopeful expectancy in the midst of sin and suffering (Rom 8:23–24). Inasmuch as the resurrection is the guarantee of Jesus' presence through the Spirit with believers now, there is nothing that can separate us now or in the future from the love of God in Christ Jesus (Rom 8:39).

While this hope offers people ground for transcending their present circumstances, it becomes a present and personal hopefulness as it is received subjectively; for it is through meaningful relationships in the community of those who hope that hope is experientially sustained. Indeed, the nurture of hope is inseparable from the loving solidarity of community, for "hope is something that we do together."[48] It is noteworthy that, in our research, references to solidarity in sustaining hope through the journey are conspicuous by their absence. It is pertinent, too, that the only reference to hope among the caregiver-participants was the bereaved partner's poignant comment that he has no hope except "the future hope," and that does not give him what he needs "to go on with" in his present grief. Had he experienced near-at-hand comfort from such a witness in the fellowship of a compassionate, sustaining, hoping community of Christ's people through the long journey, that future hope might have become present hope to sustain and lead him forward. The challenge must be issued to Christian congregations to be, as individuals and as community, mediators of Christ's compassion, comfort, and hope.

Sustaining Identity

If the Christian community is important for our sustenance in suffering and hoping, its role in sustaining our identity is no less important. As we have discussed, identity is constructed and reconstructed in relationship, and it is worth attention that the "social self" (Sabat's "Self 3") is entirely

---

47. Pembroke, *Pastoral Care*, 99–101. See also pp. 101–6 for liturgies that foster hope.
48. Ibid., 99.

dependent on others for its existence. Furthermore, with the perspective that the followers of Christ are interdependent members of the body of Christ, that "social self" has an added dimension. As our social selves are nurtured through relationship with others, so we are sustained as social *and* spiritual selves through relationship and participation in the body of Christ. Indeed, Kenneson argues that gathering is vital in sustaining life-giving connections, that it is in gathering that the ecclesia learns to receive its true identity and "confesses that there is no 'I' apart from that body: that every person receives his or her truest identity as a part of the Body of Christ."[49]

We have argued that caring for a person with dementia *begins* with the narrative of a person whose personhood is God-given and cannot be lost, a person who is held by God, who does not abandon. This beginning point is crucial. But it is as the person is "re-membered" in a community of persons-in-relation that the person's identity is *sustained*. The community becomes "a community of remembering" for the person who may forget.[50] As the body of Christ remembers, with the person and for her, who she is, her story, and her future, she is "brought back together," and sustained in who she is in Christ. Such a picture of the community's remembering presents a stark contrast with the experiences of some of those in our caregiver study. We are reminded of Beverley's assessment of their church's response to her husband: after thirty years of participation in the community, "it's almost like they fall off the edge of the earth."

But how are we, the body of Christ, to remember? What are we expecting, and what are we seeing? Do we only tell the stories of the past, of the person who served, or sang, or showed love? Do we merely look forward, to "the future hope"? No. The apostle Paul presents a metaphor from which most of us have possibly drawn reassurance at our times of weakness and frailty, the metaphor of clay pots, frail and ordinary, but holding the all-surpassing glory of God (2 Cor 4:7–10). At what point along the spectrum of mobility, or fading eyesight, or along the line of forgetting, does this frailty bring exclusion? Together, and in humility, we are called to remember that within each person in Christ resides the glory of God, now. We are reminded that we *need* one another for the sustenance of our true identity, as we "fix our eyes not on what is seen but on what is unseen" (2 Cor 4:18),

---

49. Kenneson, "Gathering," 63.
50. Swinton, *Dementia*, 221–23.

as we see, in faith, the presence of Christ, the work of the Spirit, and the glory of God in one another.

Sustaining Community

Worship and Rituals

How then, do we work at fostering a faithful, faith-filled Christian community that reflects the self-giving, sustaining love of God, and lives out the narrative of faith and hope and compassion? Making the point that gatherings play an important role in forming the social imagination and moral horizon of a group, Kenneson argues that the gathered Christian community is the embodied response to God's prior action, formed to be an embodied witness in the world to God's love for the world.[51] If an orientation toward God as the source of life and all gifts—an orientation alien to our contemporary culture—is proclaimed and enacted in our gatherings, a sense of dependence on God and one another is fostered.[52] The gathered community, through waiting on God and offering itself for God's purposes, is shaped and formed to take its place in working out God's ultimate purposes and extending God's reign in the world.[53] As we participate in the enacted meta-narrative of salvation in Christ through the sacramental life of the gathered community, the values of belonging to God and serving others are instilled, and our understanding of identity as person-in-community is developed.[54] This enactment through ritual and liturgy has a deeper impact than the merely cognitive; indeed, as Pembroke argues, with the Holy Spirit as the agent of formation, the Christian self, person-in-community, is *formed* through ritual:

> It is not that the bread, wine, water and oil *mean* something that is the crucial fact; rather it is that the performance of the ritual signs and gestures *constitutes a people* shaped by these meaning structures.... Eating bread and drinking wine together *is* community, *is* the transcendence of individualism.[55]

---

51. Kenneston, "Gathering," 55–56.
52. Ibid., 56–60.
53. Ibid., 59–66.
54. Pembroke, *Pastoral Care*, 148.
55. Ibid., 149. Italics in original text.

Thus, the sacraments, rituals, words, and gestures of the gathered people—including such physical gestures as "sharing the peace"—are formative of community.[56] (It is interesting to reflect that, with the possible exception of someone to give a welcome handshake at the door, shaking hands in "passing the peace" may offer the only physical touch or eye contact for a person attending the service alone—if this ritual is practiced.) In relation to the power of spoken and sung words in shaping community, Pembroke draws our attention to psychological research demonstrating the power of words to shape our individual or collective self.[57] In light of this, the content of our hymns and songs calls for reflection. In thumbing through the well known hymns of the past three centuries at least, and the "praise songs" of the past five decades, it is difficult not to be struck by the overwhelming focus on "I" and "mine" rather than "we" and "ours"; and in reflecting on the quite common practice of standing in rows watching a group of singers leading (or perhaps performing) the singing, with possibly minimal congregational engagement, we are challenged to explore new ways and words and actions to rebuild a sense of relational, interdependent community grounded in and motivated by the love of God, as we seek to swim against the tide of a self-focused, autonomous, and individualized culture.

Prayer

Shared intercessory prayer in the body has a role in bringing together corporate and personal elements of pastoral care. Three of the caregivers express the desire for others to pray with or for them. Participants in the pastoral practice study comment on the response of persons with advanced dementia to familiar prayers; however, there are few references to intercessory prayer. The Gospel narratives present a pattern of people pleading earnestly to Jesus on behalf of their friends, as for example Mark 2:3–12. In this narrative, presented in all the Synoptic Gospels, it is the friends' compassionate, active, expectant, and creative faith to which Jesus responds, "seeing their faith" (Mark 2:5); and the paralyzed man who has been brought to Jesus is blessed and made whole both spiritually and physically. Biblical narratives like this one highlight the responsibility of the community of faith to *be* the community of faith, to exercise compassionate, active

---

56. Ibid., 149–50.
57. Ibid., 145–48.

faith in bringing to God, together with them, the needs of those who suffer and need support.

Such prayer is a distinguishing feature of the body of Christ as it takes part in Christ's intercession (Rom 8:34), bringing people into God's outpoured blessings.[58] Johnson notes that intercessory prayer is the expression of the church where it is united in its commitment to the mind of Christ, and therefore united in its commitment to bearing each other's burdens; and she points out that where the church prays for others—for example, for the poor—as "them," somewhere away from us, we fail to be the unified, inclusive body.[59] As she says about intercessory prayer:

> To pray rightly, Christians must engage in the awkward, conflict-filled process . . . of overcoming fear and pride and self-deception to begin to know each other as members of one body. . . . The unity of the Church in liturgy, which is friendship enacted through gift-giving, requires mutuality, facing each other as peers, as family, as members of each other and therefore as constitutive of each other's well-being.[60]

Johnson adds that where such prayer is not answered in the ways pleaded for, we continue to stand together in solidarity and hope and continue to pray,[61] knowing and remembering together the larger narrative, and affirming that "he has not despised or disdained the suffering of the afflicted one; he has not hidden his face from him but has listened to his cry for help" (Ps 22: 24).

Participation in intercession is a high privilege. Not only do we participate in Christ's intercession; Paul speaks also of the Holy Spirit interceding before God for us (Rom 8:26–27), and this picture of the Spirit's intercession gives insight particularly relevant for prayer with and for persons with dementia. This is a picture of wordless prayer arising from "an inarticulate realm of human vulnerability" where God the sustaining Spirit acts within and beyond a person, interacting with the person's inner sighs and interceding at the point of deepest human confusion, sustaining the deepest levels of human consciousness and unconsciousness;[62] where the groans of suffering "are being drawn by the Spirit into . . . the glory of a dialogue

---

58. Johnson, "Praying: Poverty," 229–30.
59. Ibid., 232.
60. Ibid., 233.
61. Ibid., 234.
62. Jewett, *Romans: Commentary*, 524.

within deity itself."[63] Where words are lost, and confusion and pain and vulnerability can no longer be articulated, the community has the privilege of interceding, of being with the person before God, and participating in the activity of the Spirit. Likewise, in a one-to-one relationship with a person with dementia, "being present" takes on deeper significance in light of this picture of intercession. Not only can we expect to connect with a person "spirit to spirit," but, in light of the Holy Spirit's activity, we can have an active, expectant faith that the Spirit is present in a special way to express to the Father the unspoken yearnings of the person's depths. Intercessory prayer, then, is deeply significant in the corporate and personal aspects of pastoral care in the journey.

Contemplative Awareness

Thus a community reflects God's remembering, through people's attentiveness, empathy, their "being present" with a person. Silence may be called for in entering into solidarity with the deep suffering of others in "wordless empathy,"[64] and we have already noted the importance of a sacred space of quietness and stillness, in connecting with persons with dementia. In the noise and busyness of life in general, and of church life in particular, such qualities may be foreign. Where are the disciplines of contemplative awareness and meditation to be learnt and nurtured, if not in the context of the congregation? We need to "consciously create pools of silence in which to hear. We quiet the many voices around us and within us as we wait to hear a word of revelation."[65] Such traditions, McCarthy argues, develop and are handed down within a community that keeps them alive, and we need Christian communities that nurture us and hold us in these practices—practices that foster encounter with the sacred, and in turn, encounter with those who suffer.

Meaning-making in Community

From a ground of solidarity in suffering, communally nurtured hope, and communally sustained identity, meaning may be sought in the complexity

---

63. Ibid., 525.
64. Zylla, *Roots of Sorrow*, 88.
65. McCarthy, "Spirituality," 200.

of the dementia challenges. We have discussed the value of listening well to people's stories in the rebuilding of their identity, but the value of such listening is no less in allowing them to make sense of their present experiences in a context of loving empathy and hopeful presence. Swinton draws attention to the paradox of identity in persons with dementia, of a fragile identity dependent on others for sustenance, and a divine identity sustained by God and transcending the realities of the bodily life; and he acknowledges that "we can, and should, mourn our personal loss of memory. But if God remembers us, we are provided with a source of deep and enduring hope."[66]

What response, then, is appropriate when faced with the hard question of offering hope and sustenance on the one hand, and acknowledging the losses and validating the grief of the dementia experience on the other? Significant challenges confront those who accompany loved ones on the dementia journey: to remember and affirm the divine identity while faced with a very fragile social identity, and to deal with the apparent opposites of sustaining a loved one in hope and relationship while at the same time acknowledging their own losses and working through their own complex grief.

Drawing on the writings of Lynch, Pembroke encourages the use of the ironic imagination in order to accept the coexistence of opposites, seeing this as a valuable quality for the Christian in making meaning of life's challenges, and finding hope in suffering.[67] For the person in early dementia, such ironic imagination might foster both an assured hope in the identity that God continues to sustain *and* an acceptance of the present and future reality of loss. For caregivers, too, employing the ironic imagination might allow an acknowledgement of the changes in the loved one's self while seeing the person's identity secure in Christ. Thus, the losses might be grieved *and* the person's identity might be sustained and relationship nurtured with a joyful acceptance of occasional reappearances of the "hidden" self. For Christians facing their own diagnosis and those walking the dementia road with them, it becomes possible then to hold contraries together. Suffering and hope, loss and life, lament and love come together within the overarching narrative, the narrative that began before time in the plans of God and leads us forward through the death and resurrection of Christ into the ultimate victory over suffering and into wholeness in Christ.

66. Swinton, *Dementia*, 198.
67. Pembroke, *Pastoral Care*, 110–12.

Grounded Care

These theological perspectives ground an approach to dementia care in a supportive community of faith. Objections may be raised and inconsistencies highlighted. Such theological foundations may be sound, but is there theological articulation or practical expression of them in Christian communities? In other words, what is the use of theology and theory, if practice says something very different? As with any journey, we need to know where we are going and why; and then we move step by step from where we are to where we are going. The need and the responsibility to care are very clear. If care is theologically and practically grounded in loving Christian community, the isolation of the journey may be minimized; the grief of inevitable losses may be validated; the suffering may be expressed, heard, and eased; and valued persons may be sustained in their personhood and in hope. Thus, the narrative of individual lives may be incorporated in the meta-narrative of the faithful and compassionate God who entered into our life of suffering to bring abundant life and eschatological hope.

8

A Pastoral Approach

As we experience community as a body in which we have been called by Jesus to belong to each other, we discover that we are responsible for each others' growth and for the development of each others' gifts. We have the power to call forth the gifts of others or to crush them.
—JEAN VANIER, BROKEN BODY

WE CONFRONT THE RESPONSIBILITY of providing a Christian pastoral response that expresses the love of God to people facing the challenges of dementia in our church communities, and to those beyond who make this journey alone or unsupported. Such a response begins with fostering healthy interdependent Christian communities. From within such communities, it becomes possible to offer ongoing pastoral one-to-one relationships and support in the family context, and to establish a churches-based support program inclusive of the broader community. In this approach, we deliberately avoid any distinction between the support offered to persons with dementia and that offered to caregivers, for there are not different categories of people or of care. Each person is an individual with particular needs, gifts, and vulnerabilities; and *agape* relationships and relational skills will call forth the gifts of each, and benefit each and all together as persons-in-relationship.

Pastoral Care: Building Healthy Communities

Person-honoring Values

With the theological foundation of a personhood bestowed by God, it is to be expected that persons will be honored *particularly* in Christian communities. Within healthy Christian communities, all are respected and loved and have the opportunity to flourish in interdependence. With such values, the message will be communicated that help-giving is a joy, that we are for and with one another in community to share the load; and the independence and unwillingness to "impose" expressed by participant-caregivers will give way to an understanding that coping and help-seeking are not mutually exclusive. Indeed, where acknowledging vulnerability and asking for help are recognized as gifts rather than signs of failure, community becomes possible. In a context of interdependence, people are honored in the reciprocity of friendship, rather than care being "done to needy people" from a position of superiority; and condescending attitudes of sympathy or even pity towards aged or needy persons are banished. A person-honoring acceptance in empathic relationships will ameliorate feelings of abandonment, shame, or embarrassment in those facing the challenges of suffering, loss, forgetfulness, and aging in themselves or a loved one. Thus the malignant social psychology that produces shame, labeling, exclusion, stigma, and sheer neglect of persons with dementia will give way to a community of *agape* love, empathic understanding, affirmation, embrace, and well-being for all.

Equipping for Care

Teaching

The pastoral role in a congregation includes equipping people to care. The view that caring people are the only resource needed to provide support in the dementia journey—expressed by a local pastoral care coordinator—invites reflection, in light of the apparent gaps in pastoral practice and caregivers' experiences in their churches. Certainly, Christlike self-giving love, received and shared in the power of the Spirit, is the source of and the motive underlying the church's true pastoral ministry. Without this, no amount of training will produce genuine, mutual, loving relationships with other members of the body. Certainly, too, we need to be careful to avoid trusting in "psychosocial fads" rather than the ministry of the presence of God in the power of the Holy Spirit.[1] However, obviously something has to change in at least some contemporary congregational life if people are to be cared for well on this journey. Even with a genuine desire to express love, the powerful conditioning of a self-seeking, independent, pain-avoiding, and cognitively-based culture needs to be identified and countered. Teaching and modeling based on the theological concept of the body composed of interdependent members who need and value one another—and who especially honor the more vulnerable—will foster relationships where mutuality and compassion are called forth. Personal growth in spirituality through prayer, meditation on Scripture, and openness to the ministry of the Holy Spirit will be encouraged and will nurture self-giving relationships. Indifference and avoidance of grief and "negative" emotions will be challenged by biblical teaching about the expression of suffering and comfort in the body. A deep understanding is called for in relation to personhood, our identity in Christ, and the challenges of dementia. Where there are patronizing attitudes, they must be challenged by teaching that fosters a mutuality of care within congregations and in pastoral care teams, where "sharing with" replaces a hierarchical pastoral "doing for" others.

Fostering Empathic Relationships

In an individualistic, self-focused, and "time-poor" contemporary culture, self-giving friendship, empathy, and sensitivity to one another's needs become increasingly elusive. With the advent of potentially distancing forms of communication such as the social media and texting rather than face-to-face, voice-to-voice, touch-to-touch, and person-to-person connection, training is called for in such communication skills as active, sensitive listening, and being really present. Offering one's own space for hospitable, empathic connection with another builds and fosters self-giving relationships in community, as people set aside their own agendas and enter the world of others with attentiveness; and developing the empathic imagination deepens understanding and fuels compassion. In a busy, driven society, these skills and actions are counter-cultural, and may need to be learned and nurtured.

When skills in listening and presence are employed in relationships across the community, an empathic hospitality develops that will enable

1. Purves, *Pastoral Theology*, 207.

people to be heard and known, touched and loved as persons, rather than viewed as problems to be avoided or categories to be stigmatized, ignored, and feared. The exercise of these skills will facilitate the enfranchisement of grief, the finding of meaning, the building and rebuilding of identity, and deep friendships, rather than fleeting acquaintances in the body. Such broadening and deepening of friendship connections and hospitality will develop an inclusive community network that does not leave aged persons, persons with dementia, and caregivers stranded in isolation when friends in their cohort succumb to ill-health, changed circumstances, or relocation. These and further skills in listening such as narrative literacy—listening and co-constructing the person's personal narrative through story, art, and music—empower caring people to understand and facilitate not only verbally-articulate narratives but also non-verbal and fragmented-verbal ones, and allow the story of each person to be heard and valued, relational connection to be maintained, and a person's identity to be nurtured.

The losses and complex grief of the dementia journey call for understanding and support; and equipping people for empathic listening will facilitate not only the expression of the whole range of emotions, but also the making of meaning in the confusion of the journey. This listening is needed across the entire faith community, not merely from "pastoral specialists," but with each member doing her/his part in valuing and caring for other members of the body. (The poignancy of the references of participants in the caregiver research to other members "not wanting to know," "shutting the door," and "not understanding" drove home this need!) Such listening will guard against empathic failure in this part of a person's network, perhaps the person's *only* network, and will offer solidarity in suffering and hoping, rather than reinforcing isolation and despair. Grief will be enfranchised, allowing persons to rediscover their spiritual resources, make sense in their losses, and find meanings in their own narratives in the larger context of a historical faith narrative of God's faithfulness and God's remembering. In these ways the church will affirm its true identity as a people who love one another.

Facilitating Inclusive Worship

Accessibility to and participation in worship must be facilitated. The denial of worship opportunities to persons with dementia has been described as

A Pastoral Approach

a "grave scandal."[2] While churches may not accept a judgment of "denial of worship," the outcome is no less disturbing where stigma or the neglect of people results in their absence from corporate worship, and their disconnection and disappearance from the community of faith. Therefore, careful consideration must be given to inclusive worship accessible to people with dementia and caregivers—and to people with hearing and vision impairment and mobility challenges. There should be provision for practical needs such as transport, *offered* by the community rather than asked for by those with need. Attention needs to be given to physical accessibility and to effective sound equipment and clear articulation in all parts of worship services, to minimize the sense of exclusion or frustration of people seeking sustenance in their faith amid life's challenges.

Worship services should be offered that take account of the needs of the elderly and those with cognitive impairment. In light of the significance of rituals and practices that foster continuity with the past and connection with God, others, and the self, it is worth reflecting on current practices. In congregations that are less sacramental or more informal in their approach to worship, the changes of the recent past may have been considerable: the changes in music style, volume, instruments, and language; changes in the sacrament of Holy Communion format and in the administering of the elements and the level of formality, with a shift toward informality and the elimination of familiar liturgy; changes in the wording of the Lord's prayer; and, for many, changes in the atmosphere, from varying degrees of solemnity, quietness, and reflection to informality, laughter, noise, and busyness. For a person with dementia whose early memories come to the fore, this may feel like a very alien environment. An awareness of and a sensitivity to the needs of *all* generations and conditions of members of the body should be fostered. The inclusion of meaningful liturgies and times of quietness and meditation in regular worship services will acknowledge the needs of those who may be struggling, and may develop a compassionate awareness in those who are not.[3] Scripture-based teaching concerning suffering, grief, compassion, and the body will enlarge people's assumptive world to include the challenges of life and the interdependence of all—with the added benefit of preparing *all* for the possibility of unexpected and "unfair" suffering. Intercessory prayers and psalms of lament might integrate the experience

---

2. Shamy, *Spiritual Dimension*, 95.

3. For example, Pembroke, *Pastoral Care*, 164–65 offers a "litany of love," for fostering a love ethic.

of suffering into the larger narrative of faith, acknowledge and validate the emotions, and encourage a sense of solidarity with one another in suffering.

As well, midweek services might be offered, in a style familiar and appropriate for those who do not function well in fast-paced noise and unfamiliarity. Persons in earlier dementia may be willing and able to contribute in such a setting, through participation in music, reading, or creative arts.[4] Such services might also facilitate the attendance of caregivers through providing in-home relational care for their loved one if no longer able to participate. If participation in worship services becomes impossible, connection should be maintained through home visiting where "sacred presence," prayer, and the sacrament of Holy Communion are shared regularly. By all means, in a healthy community there will be serious attention to welcoming, embracing, and being with and for one another, with gladness.

Pastoral Care: Companions

For caregivers *and* persons with dementia, the care of a pastoral companion on the journey should complement that of a supportive community. The needs of a person facing the challenges of cognitive loss firsthand have been articulated with deep insight by Christine Bryden, across many years of the journey. Bryden, in acknowledging the vital importance of her spirituality and the need for sensitive help in connecting with her faith, speaks for others as well as herself. While initially struggling with retaining a sense of who she is, she later affirms that her spiritual relationship with God through Christ is an important and increasing source of identity, and that "my spirit is me and always will be me."[5] In creating a "new sense of becoming," she notes the need to find meaning in the suffering and thus to overcome the fear of the losses. She acknowledges the value of spiritual guidance and direction throughout the journey, and the importance of care partnerships rather than care being done to the person.[6] The value of a spiritual director or companion has already been noted, a person who listens with openness and love, in the crisis of identity and meaning that may confront a person throughout this spiritual journey. Caregivers also need such a listener: participants in the caregiver study clearly articulated their

---

4. McFadden, "Creative Expression," 105–6.
5. Bryden, *Dancing with Dementia*, 158.
6. MacKinlay, *Creating Care*, 45.

longing for someone who would listen with understanding, and indicated (in some cases graphically) the impacts of traveling alone.

In the complexity of the loss on this journey, a trained pastoral companion will offer opportunities for the person to process grief and make meaning in the context of the person's belief system. Spiritual reminiscence with a companion might allow persons, both those with dementia and caregivers and where possible both together, to reflect on spiritual memories and the present faith journey, to sustain the identity of the person with forgetfulness, to find meaning, and to experience growth rather than diminution of their faith and identity. Such a companion will listen to the ongoing narrative, enter the person's suffering, facilitate the expression of emotions, be the faithful witness to hope, and intercede in prayer. Shared psalms of lament, prayer, and rituals developed together for significant occasions might acknowledge the ongoing grief. Such occasions might include the time of diagnosis, significant milestones in the life and relationship of the person/s (such as wedding anniversaries), and particularly around the time of entry into a residential aged care center. At this time, in light of the distress of caregiver-partners, the wedding vows might be reaffirmed and "reframed" to encourage acceptance of a new era of commitment, caring, and oneness, in place of feelings of guilt and "betrayal" of the vows. The spiritual companion's ongoing support for the caregiver *and* the person during the person's time in the residential aged care center "re-members" the person in the Christian community rather than "dismembering the body," allows both to remain connected as part of the church community, and maintains a supportive connection into the time of bereavement. In these ways, the complex and often long grief of the journey is acknowledged and processed in love, faithfulness, and hope; and the depths of suffering are shared.

A spiritual companion will actively nurture identity throughout the journey. A one-to-one relationship that offers empathy through deep, imaginative listening allows a person to rebuild her identity and discover meaning in the losses and in life. The spiritual companion might encourage a person in early dementia to recall the "sparkling moments" of life, past and present, to enjoy them and incorporate them into the counter-story of life in the midst of challenge, and to nurture the personal identity.[7] With the gradual loss of coherent verbal communication, the sparkling moments can still be recalled by the companion, with joy and understanding. For the caregiver, speaking of these moments of joy and connection with the loved

---

7. Pembroke, *Renewing Practice*, 62–63.

one will assist in building and holding the positive aspects of the journey, and in remembering and affirming the relationship and who the loved one is. The companion might also enlist the aid of a "nurturing third" person from the friendship network to foster the counter-story of meaningful shared experiences.[8]

Journeying as a companion will mean being there throughout. Where the companion's relationship is ongoing with the person with dementia, the loss of verbal skills will be merely a transition in ways of connecting, rather than a loss of relationship. Such one-to-one deep connection invites a waiting expectancy in a welcoming space between, and the indwelling Holy Spirit who "links our souls, our spirits, not our minds or brains"[9] continues to intercede for and be with the person, the absence of words notwithstanding—and the connection is indeed sacred. For the caregiver also, the companion will be there in the journey through grief towards hope and meaning at distressing transitions, and if the caregiver is no longer recognized. When the loved one dies, the complex grief will be ameliorated by the continuing comfort of the faithful witness to the God who has not abandoned.

Pastoral Care: Advocacy

Advocacy is acknowledged to be integral to the pastoral role. In light of the isolation, burden, and grief that may accompany dementia, community support services must be enhanced. The literature on supportive person-centered care, research indicating the value of spirituality for well-being, and the employment of spiritual strategies for coping indicate the value of spiritual care in improving the quality of life and wellbeing of persons with dementia and caregivers across the whole community, including those of all faith traditions and those who profess no faith. Advocacy will be at several levels.

Advocacy in the Community

The scope of spiritual care should be extended into our social structures and systems, affirming that spiritual care is an important aspect of

---

8. Ibid., 64–65.
9. Bryden, *Dancing with Dementia*, 74.

whole-person care that may bring peace, hope, connectedness, and meaning. A case might be presented to community care providers, Alzheimer's organizations, and all levels of government for funding that acknowledges the emotional and spiritual as well as the social and practical needs on the dementia journey. Home visits from professional spiritual caregivers should be at least as accessible as medical or social care for all those on the journey, where they can receive regular support. This is particularly valuable at times of heightened stress such as around diagnosis, placement in aged care centers, and during the late palliative stage; and spiritual care is an important aspect of holistic care for aged care center residents including those with dementia. On this journey, such care might significantly reduce the impacts of grief and stress, and ameliorate the spiritual pain and distress of the most difficult periods and aspects of the journey. In light of the acknowledged importance of spiritual connections for persons *throughout* the dementia journey, advocacy will underline the value of spiritual care, including one-to-one connection in pastoral relationships.

Advocacy in the Church

Running counter to an individualistic, task-oriented, and fragmented society, there is a unique element in Christian community as we are drawn into and bound together by Christ's life. The biblical testimony, affirmed by virtually all theological ethicists, is that God has a fundamental option for the poor and the oppressed; and care that acknowledges the value of all people, especially the vulnerable and the stranger, witnesses to divine grace and love. Inclusive friendship offers the possibility of revealing something of God through reflecting Jesus' model of loving the stranger as a neighbor, in a world where all are neighbors. Where these biblical values are not expressed, acted upon, and prized in church communities, advocacy is essential.

The health of congregations and individuals being inseparable, church leaders should be strongly encouraged to preach and foster values such as those of 1 Corinthians 12 and 13, and to offer worship services that reflect a particular awareness of the needs of the suffering and aging as well as the young and happy, thus honoring them as integral and valued members of Christian community. Pastoral care coordinators might advocate for church services as described above, acknowledging the value of all members. Advocacy may be needed for the provision of appropriate worship services in aged care centers for churches' own members and any other residents who wish to connect or reconnect with God.

Broadening the Care: Interchurch Program

The threads of theology, theory, research, and practice elaborated in this work are drawn together to facilitate a supportive context for those facing the challenges of dementia. An initiative is proposed, the establishment of an inter-church program, to offer caring supportive friendship for church members, and to extend this friendship to people in the wider community. Employing informed pastoral leaders and trained volunteers from across local congregations and from within the community, a place of spiritual and emotional sustenance and friendship for both persons with dementia and caregivers might be created in a church facility, with an invitation extended to all local churches *and* to any persons experiencing the challenges of dementia in the wider community.

Participation

In planning the establishment of such an inter-church and community program, the value of solidarity is recognized through the sharing of gifts and resources across Christian congregations and in the local community. *All* local churches in an area should be invited to participate in such a program, both through the provision of volunteers and the promotion of the program for those on the dementia journey. Advocacy at this interchurch level might include information to enhance understanding of the challenges of those facing the dementia journey and the value of long-term emotional and spiritual support. The local government authority should be included in communications, to explain the purposes and proposed structure of the program and to seek support. Appropriate publicity in the wider community would be necessary, and community care service providers might be contacted and encouraged to promote this support program among their clients facing the challenges of dementia.

Structure

Monthly Program

The proposed program includes a range of supportive gatherings each month and across the year. A *caregivers'* support group might meet once a month, oriented to addressing participants' emotional and spiritual needs, with volunteers available to provide respite care for their loved ones with dementia. Similarly, a monthly support group might be established (during a second week of the month) for *persons with dementia*, particularly early in their journey.

In each of these groups, with facilitative leadership, there would be a variety of activities throughout a year, including social and creative activities, and the sharing of memories, life narratives, and spiritual reminiscence. Such sharing would facilitate engagement in the meaning-making process in the often confusing journey, and allow this part of the life journey to be integrated into the person's whole life narrative and, where appropriate, a broader faith narrative. The processing of emotional and spiritual pain, ambiguous loss, and grief would be facilitated in a context of mutuality and empathy. Space should be provided for laughter and light relief, together with opportunities in the caregivers group for sharing insights into the life-story of the loved one and the current challenges; and there might also be input on means of dealing with stress and grief. Fun and food should always be included—to offer hospitality, encourage friendship-building, and reduce stress. The differing needs of caregivers and persons with dementia might thus be supported by others who face the challenges specific to their perspective. For persons with dementia, their group would provide opportunities to give as well as receive care, to develop social connections, and to maintain their social identity in a supportive environment. The training and participation of volunteers from churches and the community would deepen the understanding of these helpers, build meaningful, compassionate connections, and eliminate stigma.

A monthly morning tea for *persons with dementia and their caregivers together* might be provided in another week of the month. This would offer continuing supportive social contact and relationship-building; and the maintenance and rebuilding of couple-identity would be facilitated for partners. Again, the involvement of volunteers in a serving capacity would build connections and enhance their empathy for those on the journey.

A monthly friendship lunch might be provided for any older people in the churches and the wider community, where isolation and loneliness would be lessened in a context of friendship. Such a regular event would be instrumental in maintaining an inclusive social network, developing friendships, and breaking down barriers of stigma and fear. Meaningful friendships in such a group would allow people to express their concerns and fears about memory loss, and these supportive, trustworthy connections would reduce the possibility that people facing memory loss would disappear unnoticed from their social network.

Shared Worship

To complement this monthly program, a quarterly worship service might be established, with program participants and other members of congregations leading segments of the service where possible. Such corporate worship should be accessible and relevant, through the development of liturgies that acknowledge the challenges of aging, suffering, grief, and dementia. The appropriate use of movement and touch, such as "the passing of the peace" might be employed. Times of quietness, peaceful music, pictures of natural beauty, and a slower pace might accommodate the preferences of participants in the program.

Grief Enfranchised

Finally, an annual memorial service might be offered, to support the bereaved. This would further enfranchise this complex grief, encouraging the expression of emotions through the sensitive use of rituals honoring those who have died, and offering hope in suffering to those who grieve. Other members of church congregations should be invited to participate in these services, thus offering solidarity with those facing the challenges of loss and aging.

The emotional and spiritual challenges of the journey are thus supported, interdependence is fostered, the "invisibility" of those on the journey is reduced, grief is enfranchised during the journey and following a loved one's death, and self-giving and mutuality of caring are encouraged. Thus, *agape* love is expressed, reducing isolation and transforming strangers into friends.

A Responsive Approach

In summary, such a pastoral care model responds to the needs of those facing the challenges of dementia, individually and together, within Christian congregations and in the wider community. Grounded in the theology and fellowship of the church and drawing on research and theory from cultural sources, it offers a practical means of enhancing awareness and acceptance, and sustaining persons in the name and the love of Christ. It acknowledges the relational roles, responsibilities, and interdependence of congregational members as sharers in and of the love of God; and it facilitates the development of places of acceptance, friendship, prayer, and belonging, both for members of local churches and for those in the wider community. In acknowledgment of the crucial importance of sustaining personhood and identity through ongoing relationships, opportunities are created for relationships with others facing similar challenges, and with companions who listen with imaginative empathy in one-to-one ongoing relationship. Thus, those on the journey have opportunity to build a narrative of their experience in the context of their whole life narrative and a larger narrative of faith. Where there is confusion about the meaning of the experience, or spiritual pain in attempting to reconcile global and situational meaning, there are opportunities for talking to make sense, find benefit, and receive support in drawing on spiritual as well as cognitive and emotional resources. Mutuality of care is fostered in Christian communities; pastoral companions are available for the journey; and in support groups the value and dignity of each person is acknowledged in giving as well as receiving. Grief is validated and supported corporately and individually, and the community offers solidarity in suffering and hoping. The faithful, hospitable, ongoing presence of individual people in supportive Christian communities thus expresses something of the qualities of the Triune God, reaching out gladly to all persons with the love from which even the dementia journey cannot separate them.

9

Moving Forward

*Dear children, let us not love with words or tongue
but with actions and in truth.*
—1 John 3:18.

Taking Stock

Dementia presents a social issue of significant dimensions in a hypercognitive culture where stigma, negative stereotyping, and societal isolation accompany forgetfulness. This issue raises serious theological, ecclesiological, and pastoral questions that call for a response from the Christian community, and within the field of practical theology, we seek to address these questions. We learn what we can about the phenomenon from cultural sources and from "on-the-ground" research; and from here, through theological reflection, we work to develop Christian pastoral practice that addresses the gaps and silences in theory and practice, and expresses the relational love of God flowing into and within the Christian community and overflowing to a hurting world.

In confronting this pastoral question, in essence we have sought to answer the questions *to whom, why,* and *how*. Firstly, then, we have sought to establish *who* is to be sustained. Particularly in light of the commonly expressed or implied view of persons with dementia as "lost persons," this is a vital question. In dementia studies within the social sciences, we have seen that the foundation of person-centered and supportive care approaches is an understanding of persons as essentially relational, their personhood bestowed by other persons in relationship; and much care focuses on building environments where relationships are nurtured. From a trinitarian theological perspective we have found common ground, in that relationship is at the core of our being as persons. However, we go further, arguing for an inviolable personhood bestowed by God, that includes both the vertical dimension of relationship with a personal, loving, relating God who draws persons into relationship, and the horizontal dimension of loving relationships with other persons. A theological understanding of embodied personhood sees all aspects of living, including the physical, emotional, social, and spiritual, as intrinsically connected; and this has significant implications for care that embraces whole persons in their relational context.

The spiritual dimension, infusing all areas of life, has been argued to be an important and possibly *the key* channel for connection for and with persons whose cognition has deteriorated. Such an understanding challenges bio-psychosocial models of care that stop short of including the spiritual dimension. On the other hand, the care that is advocated in dementia studies and evidenced in best practice—respectful, relational, communicative care offered in a supportive environment—challenges Christian communities to look at the quality of their community life and the expression of their relational care for those on the dementia journey.

For whom, then, should we, as Christians and Christian communities, care? We have both privilege and responsibility, being called to reflect the *agape* love of the Triune God and the supernaturally created unity and interdependence of a body where all in Christ belong to one another, and vulnerable members are especially honored. Within the body of Christ, each member is an essential and valued part of the body and all are called to love one another. All are called to suffer with those who suffer, and rejoice with those who rejoice; and all are called to care for and offer hospitality to the stranger, who is also the neighbor. In Jesus' words, we hear that friendship shared with the stranger and the vulnerable is offered to Jesus himself, and a withholding of love from the needy is a withholding of love from Jesus. So we are called to care: to love, honor, and sustain one another, and to recognize and value one another's story and gifts—and this "one another" includes those who travel the road of forgetting and those who travel with them.

Why should we care? From the theological ground of God's remembering, holding each person in God's own memory, we in the body of Christ are called to embody that remembering. We recognize that persons with dementia are contingent, relational body-soul persons—as are we all—sustained and remembered in relationship; and we recognize that they increasingly *depend*, in fact, on others for the sustenance of their identity. We discover that the journey into forgetfulness is likely to be an isolating, lonely, grief-ridden, and frightening one, especially so if others devalue, stigmatize, ignore, and withdraw. We acknowledge that we, the body of Christ, live in and have access to an inexhaustible source of *agape* love, and that we are called to live out that love, especially to the vulnerable in the body and beyond.

We have heard the stories of several caregivers, stories revealing not only courageous coping but also, sometimes very graphically, burden, stress, isolation, and loss. We have heard a common refrain among caregiver partners, a yearning to talk with a companion who understands; and we infer from some of the stories the indifference and neglect of Christian communities within which they journey. Without opportunities for sharing their narrative to make sense of the journey, come to terms with the losses, and nourish their loved ones' identity and their own, their journeys have been accompanied by confusion, anger, frustration, loneliness, depression, and unidentified grief and sorrow. This is the environment their loved ones inhabit. We have heard spiritual need expressed in a longing for a supportive, empathic, praying companion or community; and for some, that unmet longing has become the spiritual pain of disconnection and existential loneliness. At times the ambiguous and generally unidentified grief of these caregivers is almost palpable, and the spiritual pain and despair almost overwhelming—and we remember that we are called to care.

Our exploration of grief has given us some understanding of the loss and pain of the journey, in all its complexity of holding on and letting go, of losing and sustaining. We reflect on the stories of caregivers who long to tell their story, to make sense of the journey, and to remember who they are, and who their loved one is—but find no one to listen. We are reminded that persons with memory loss also have a bewildering journey to make sense of, and a story to tell that sustains them in who they are—but they, too, may have no one who listens and tries to understand, no one who remembers with and for them. We realize that listening, real listening, takes effort, and calls for stepping out of our world and into their world to relate to them and share their pain; and we remember that we follow one who stepped out of his world and into ours to relate to us, to share our pain, to give us life.

We have heard of the pastoral practices and attitudes of leaders and pastoral care teams in a particular area, and we ask ourselves about the practices and attitudes in *our* communities toward those on this journey, and whether there is any thought of this being a journey shared within *our* church community. We note what appears to be a widespread lack of interest among church leaders concerning pastoral issues of aging, suffering, and grief, and we ask ourselves how well equipped are our people, indeed are we ourselves, to face these issues when they confront us. We reflect theologically on our churches' corporate worship practices and our pastoral training courses and our church committee discussions—and we realize, perhaps, that we must *learn* how to care.

Loving in Action

So how should we care? We realize that we need to build and sustain healthy Christian communities, where all are valued and each belongs to all, where biblical teaching acknowledges the reality of suffering and the shared basis of hoping; and where those who suffer can give voice to their suffering and those who do not suffer, hearing, will weep with those who do. Such communities then become places of prayer and comfort and solidarity in suffering, and an authentic witness to the power, presence, and compassion of God in the complexities of life. Such communities become places of belonging, where the narrative of the individual may be integrated into the larger narrative of faith; and where the personhood of each person, given and sustained first by God, is nourished and affirmed in relationships among friends. And such communities become places of welcome and hospitality as we reach out with the love of God to those beyond our doors who face spiritual distress, who suffer and are alone.

So we work toward sustaining persons grieving losses. We address the need for a supportive context at the church level through education, advocacy, and corporate worship practices that build flourishing, interdependent, empathic community. We go further, addressing the need for grief support and ongoing emotional and spiritual connection and nourishment by training empathic companions to listen throughout the journey; and we initiate an inter-church program that addresses the social, spiritual, and relational needs of those in the dementia journey. We do so through providing opportunities that encourage mutuality in relationship, meaning-making, identity building, and creativity, and so we reach out to those in the wider community with the inclusive love of God.

And, in humility and with the awareness that we ourselves have failed to care adequately for embodied, relational, valued persons, we advocate for holistic care throughout the journey for *all*, those of all faith traditions and those whose spirituality is expressed outside of established religions, those who are forgetting and those who journey with them. We offer our contribution towards dementia care, underlining the need for systemic change in community healthcare and residential aged care to include spiritual and emotional support as well as practical and social services for the dementia journey, both for caregivers and persons with dementia, in their own homes and in aged care centers. We draw attention to the need for care that addresses the pervasive stress, ongoing grief, increasing isolation, and changing identity of caregivers, for their own sake and to enhance the environment of the persons they care for. We affirm that spiritual caregiving offers empathic listening that might allow the expression and enfranchisement of grief and reduce the isolation and suffering; listening that might facilitate the nurture and reconstruction of the identity of caregivers and their loved ones with dementia, affirm the present qualities and personhood of the person, and foster the counter-story of life in the midst of loss. Such compassionate listening might build meaningful relationships with both caregivers and persons with dementia, and be available in times of crisis and intense grief. Ongoing support of this kind might thus ease the emotional and spiritual burden, and facilitate meaning-making in what is potentially a journey of ambiguous loss, chronic sorrow, disenfranchised grief, spiritual pain, and existential loneliness. We argue that persons with dementia have a right to emotional and spiritual nurture into the late stages of cognitive decline, and that the spiritual dimension may offer them connection with themselves, their past, others, and the transcendent, a connection possibly otherwise not accessible; and so we advocate for spiritual care in residential aged care centers.

The hope is that this model might be reflected upon, used, and refined, and extended to support those who feel alone, abandoned, or invisible on other difficult life journeys. Many other people and their family caregivers face the challenges of vulnerable mental health, chronic illness, and physical and intellectual impairment, often very long and sorrowful journeys. In an individualistic, success-oriented culture they may face similar challenges of isolation and loneliness, stigma, loss of identity, disenfranchised grief, and empathic failure that significantly affect their quality of life. A broadened inter-church program might provide support for all people confronting these challenges.

This theology-in-action addresses a serious issue of social justice, namely the needs of a sector of contemporary society at risk of being marginalized. Grounded in theological reflection on the nature and call of the Trinitarian God, the model offers the churches a tool in moving toward a transformative practice that expresses the inclusive, relational love and compassion of God, both within its own community and in its mission in the world.

Our Call

The question "what is the Christian church called to be and to do?" must be addressed repeatedly, in different eras, different contexts, different circumstances. We are called into community, we are baptized and incorporated into Christ's body, we are called to live in and live out of God's compassionate love-and-faithfulness, and we are called to embody that love and compassion on this earth, at this time. A caring, interdependent church culture includes and especially honors the vulnerable. The challenge to further develop such a culture confronts us: to build flourishing communities within which the vulnerable, the aged, the grieving, and indeed *all* are effectively included, sustained, and encouraged in mutual caring; and to reach out to the lonely and suffering with the love and compassion of God.

How then do we as Christian community and as pastoral caregivers address this particular challenge of sustaining persons grieving losses? What we cannot do is stand at a distance and avert our eyes, or bustle by on the other side of the gathered community, or excuse our indifference or blindness by believing that "those people," both persons with dementia and caregivers, are "not there," until they are no longer in our midst. We cannot stand just a little closer and pray for "them, out there," and assure them (or ourselves) that God is their comforter who will never leave them. Rather, in love we must come close. We are called to journey *together* in listening, compassionate, empathic, affirming relationship, in community that proclaims the love of our saving and compassionate God; to suffer in solidarity in one another's suffering and add our tears to one another's tears; to sit with one another in silence as mother, brother, daughter, friend, and allow our hands and our lives to touch, and together in Christ's name, receive his touch; and together, in our grief and in our hope, in God's love and one another's, we are *all* sustained.

Epilogue

GRIEF, WITH MANY FACES—USUALLY indistinct, blurred, invisible, ambiguous—may lurk beneath the surface of a family member's journey with a loved one through dementia. Sometimes the submerged and seeping emotions burst forth unbidden. This poem was my experience of grief—my only articulated grief on the long journey, though no one was there to listen. It poured out onto the page when I arrived home from a visit to my mother. If I had understood as I now understand (a couple of decades later), my thoughts and feelings may have been very different. But they were as they were.

Goodbye, My Mother

Will I recognize her today, among the half dozen white heads
    and the empty eyes?
Will her eyes, that brilliant blue, that last clue
    to her faded identity—will they be blue, dim, lost in sleep, lost . . . ?
Will there be a glimmer of life, recognition, sight?

But no—I am no longer her daughter, not her "friend," not even "lady"
. . . no longer anything to her.
Yes, I recognize her—sad and hollow eyes, sunken cheeks—
by the dress she wore last week,
the dress I bought last year, last Mothers Day,
when she still enjoyed "bright colors, pretty colors,"
    when she still knew my face . . .
    when she still enjoyed . . .
    when she still . . .

I tell them as I feed her—I tell the nurse—
"Yes, she used to cook... apple pie, egg custard, ginger sponge..."
I tell them.
"Oh yes, of course,"—with kindly concealed detachment, unbelief.
And how could they believe? I almost disbelieve myself.
    This shadow is not that person.
    This is not that.
I want to shout "She used to cook, she used to sew, she used to work, she used to live,
    she used to love. This was my mother!"
But I smile instead. I admire them. I love them for their care for her.

And anyway, I can't remember really, when she was who she was.

When did I begin forgetting, Mother, who you were?
When did *I* begin forgetting?
When should I have taken the last photo, recorded the last meaningful sentence?
When did you leave this shrunken frail shell,
    leave only this will that clutches, white knuckled,
    what is left of life?
    (and what *is* left of life?)

It is lonely here,
    holding your hand, stroking your forehead,
    trying to remember...
    clutching at threads of who you were.
Lonely there, my mother?
    Or has even that pain of living
    been lost to you?

When did you begin forgetting? Fifteen years ago?
A long time. A long time to forget—or to remember.
When, along the line of fading being, did you leave?
    When did your memory slip, beyond retrieving?
    When did your personality flicker its last, and die?
    When did you leave, my mother, when?

Epilogue

When should I have said "Goodbye, I love you, goodbye"?
When should I have grieved, cried out, sobbed my loss . . .
When, bereft, should I have sought comfort?
When should I have prayed my last prayer with you . . .
    Put a rose on the sheet,
    written the eulogy,
    committed your spirit to your Maker and your Savior?
When did you cease to be—here?
When did you leave, Mother, without goodbye?
    And why?

Goodbye, my mother, I love you. Goodbye.

Appendix A

Flexible guidelines for focused conversational interview with a caregiver

Background information; diagnosis experience and support offered

- What is your relationship with the person with dementia? For what length of time have you been caring for the person?
- How was the diagnosis communicated? How long ago? At that time, what information was given to you about the condition?
- What support was offered at that time, or what information was given about available support? By whom was the information given?
- What were your feelings then?

Losses and challenges since diagnosis

- What was life like before your loved one's dementia, and what were your hopes for the future? What has changed? What losses have there been? How are you going emotionally?
- How have you found communication with your loved one in dementia? What means of communicating have you found useful? What ways have you found of maintaining connection? Any frustrations in caring for your loved one?
- Have you experienced loneliness? Have you felt isolated? If so, how has this been? If not, where/how have the connections been maintained?

Appendix A

- What social challenges have you had? Have you felt that your loved one and/or you have been stigmatized, treated unkindly, excluded socially? If so, how has this been for you?
- Have there been any encouragements/disappointments/hurts for you in the area of emotional/spiritual support?
- What have been the main challenges for you in the experience of your loved one's dementia? What joys have there been?
- What has been the worst part of the journey?

Emotional/spiritual support in the journey so far

- What emotional and/or spiritual support have you asked for (family, friends, external agencies, other)? What has been the response?
- What support has been offered?
- How helpful or otherwise has the support been?
- What emotional/spiritual support have you been aware of that you have not accessed?
- What would have made it accessible/attractive to you?
- Who have you been able to talk to about the struggles/changes/your feelings? How was that?
- What emotions have you experienced? How and where have you expressed them? When have you felt understood or connected to someone, during this experience? How has it happened?
- What support have you needed that has not been available?

Emotional and spiritual support now and for the future

- What do you need now, in order to cope well emotionally and/or spiritually?
- What support are you receiving for these needs?
- What relationships are important to you now in this dementia experience? Why?
- Any fears/hopes about the present/future journey?

Appendix A

Emotional/spiritual support for your loved one with dementia

- What emotional and/or spiritual support has your loved one received? In what ways do you think this has been helpful? In what ways unhelpful?
- What emotional and/or spiritual support would you like your loved one with dementia to receive?

Purpose, meaning, strength, spirituality

- What has kept you going? What has given you strength? How have you coped?
- What is life about for you? What gives/has given it meaning? What do you like most about life?
- What sense/meaning, if any, do you make of your present situation, your loved one's condition? What keeps you going now?
- Have you had any experience of God/a "higher power'" in your life? What has that meant to you? How important have your beliefs/faith been to you in the past? How important now?

Religious/spiritual connections

- Are you/have you been a part of a Christian/other religious community? If so, what has been its connection with you in this journey? What support has been offered? How has this helped you or been unhelpful?
- What effects have your faith/God/guiding principles had in the experience of dementia?
- What effects has the experience had on your understanding or experience of God/faith/guiding principles?
- What place has prayer had (if any) in your experience of dementia?

Appendix A

The positive aspects of the journey

- What have you learnt/are you hoping to learn in this journey? What are the positive aspects of this experience? What are your hopes?
- Would you like to make any other comments/suggestions about your caregiving journey or your loved one's experience of dementia?

Appendix B: Local Practice Study

Appendix B.1: Email to local church leaders

Greetings,

I am engaged in a research project relating to pastoral care for persons with Alzheimer's disease or other forms of dementia and their family carers. As an important part of this project, I am exploring how pastoral care is being given to persons on the dementia journey by Christian churches in the . . . area, and what the values and challenges are in this area of ministry.

I am seeking this information via small focus groups (four or five participants) of local ministers or church pastoral care coordinators. The participants in each group meet once for approximately one hour, to share their insights, ideas, and experiences. (I am attaching a summary of the issues to be discussed.)

This research is being conducted within a PhD project in practical theology at the University of . . . and in accordance with their ethical standards. I have been working part-time on the project for three years, and have done in-depth study of relevant literature on dementia and research methods. Research work with family carers is well underway.

I have worked as a chaplain in the . . . area for the past eleven years, and have been very aware of the needs and challenges in this area of ministry.

I would really value your input or that of your pastoral care coordinator on your church's behalf, as we together seek to bring God's compassion and grace into the lives of vulnerable people.

I will contact you/your church office by phone within the next fortnight concerning your involvement, or if you prefer, you may reply by email. If you would like further information, please contact me by email: . . . or phone . . . (details provided).

Appendix B: Local Practice Study

Further information will be provided via an information and consent form prior to participation.

Yours sincerely,

Appendix B: Local Practice Study

B.2 Discussion topics for focus groups

Ongoing pastoral response to members/adherents with dementia and primary caregivers

- What experience have you had with members of your congregation who have dementia or who are caring for someone with dementia?
- What pastoral care is/has been provided for persons with dementia and for their caregivers in the congregation?
- What are the challenges in providing pastoral care for the person with dementia and in providing pastoral care for the caregiver? What do you see as the pastoral needs of each?
- What contact has been maintained with members with dementia who have gone into aged care centers/nursing homes?
- Does your congregation have involvement in church services for people with dementia in aged care centers? How does this work?

The church's response to dying persons with dementia and to caregivers

- What support has been given to the person with dementia in the late palliative stage of life? And to the family of the person?
- What bereavement support is/has been given following the death of the person with dementia? How has this worked?

Teaching/preaching on grief

- Does your church give teaching/preaching on the themes of loss and grief? What themes are addressed? How and how often?

Theology and the person with dementia

- What Scriptures/theology do you find relevant to persons with dementia? To grief?

Appendix B: Local Practice Study

Resources

- What resources have you found helpful in giving insight into the emotional and spiritual needs of the person with dementia?

Equipping the church

- In what ways could your pastoral care team and/or congregation be assisted in the provision of pastoral care to persons with dementia and their family caregivers? E.g., printed information, education, workshop, discussions, other

Anything else you would like to add on this topic

- Are there any other issues you feel are important in relation to pastorally supporting persons with dementia and their family caregivers?

Bibliography

Adams, Kathryn Betts, et al. "Personal Losses and Relationship Quality in Dementia Caregiving." *Dementia* 7.3 (2008) 301–19.
Ageing: Report of the Social Policy Committee of the Board for Social Responsibility. London: Church House, 1990.
Allan, Kate, and John Killick. "Communicating with People with Dementia." In *Supportive Care for the Person with Dementia*, edited by Julian C. Hughes et al., 217–25. Oxford: Oxford University Press, 2010.
Allen, Brian. "Remembering the Cost—A Theological Reflection." In *Between Remembering and Forgetting: The Spiritual Dimensions of Dementia*, edited by James Woodward, 6–16. London: Mowbray, 2010.
———. "Sounding the Depths: A Reflection on the Challenge of Dementia to Religious Belief and Practice." In *Spirituality and Personhood in Dementia*, edited by Albert Jewell, 153–64. London: Kingsley, 2011.
Allford, Judith. "A Relative's Perspective." In *Between Remembering and Forgetting: The Spiritual Dimensions of Dementia*, edited by James Woodward, 17–34. London: Mowbray, 2010.
Anderson, Ray S. *On Being Human: Essays in Theological Anthropology*. Grand Rapids: Eerdmans, 1982.
———. *Spiritual Caregiving as Secular Sacrament: A Practical Theology for Professional Caregivers*. London: Kingsley, 2003.
Australian Institute of Health and Welfare. *Dementia in Australia*, Cat. No. AGE 70. Canberra: AIHW, 2012.
Baldwin, Clive. "Narrative, Supportive Care, and Dementia: A Preliminary Exploration." In *Supportive Care for the Person with Dementia*, edited by Julian C. Hughes et al., 245–52. Oxford: Oxford University Press, 2010.
———. "Personhood, Personalism and Dementia: A Journey of Becoming." In *Spirituality and Personhood in Dementia*, edited by Albert Jewell, 186–97. London: Kingsley, 2011.
Barth, Karl. *Church Dogmatics*, Vol. III, Part 2. Edited by G. W. Bromiley and T. F. Torrance. Edinburgh: T. & T. Clark, 1960.
Bender, Michael. *Explorations in Dementia: Theoretical and Research Studies into the Experience of Remediable and Enduring Cognitive Losses*. London: Kingsley, 2003.
Boden, Christine. *Who Will I Be When I Die?* Sydney: Harper Collins, 1998.
Boss, Pauline. *Ambiguous Loss: Learning to Live with Unresolved Grief*. Cambridge: Harvard University Press, 1999.

Bibliography

———. *Loss, Trauma, and Resilience: Therapeutic Work with Ambiguous Loss.* New York: Norton, 2006.

Boss, Pauline, et al. "Grief in the Midst of Ambiguity and Uncertainty: An Exploration of Ambiguous Loss and Chronic Sorrow." In *Grief and Bereavement in Contemporary Society: Bridging Research and Practice*, edited by Raymond A. Neimeyer et al., 163–76. New York: Routledge Taylor & Francis, 2011.

Bramble, Marguerite, et al. "Seeking Connection: Family Care Experiences Following Long-term Dementia Care Placement." *Journal of Clinical Nursing* 18 (2009) 3118–25.

Brennan, Tim. "A Message of Love." In *Perspectives: A Newsletter for Individuals with Alzheimer's*, edited by Lisa Snyder, 4.2, 7. 1999.

Brueggemann, Walter. *Theology of the Old Testament: Testimony, Dispute, Advocacy.* Minneapolis: Fortress, 1997.

Bryden, Christine, with Sarah Minns. *Before I Forget.* Melbourne: Penguin, 2015.

Bryden, Christine. *Dancing with Dementia: My Story of Living Positively with Dementia.* London: Kingsley, 2005.

Bryden, Christine, and Elizabeth MacKinlay. "Dementia—A Spiritual Journey towards the Divine: A Personal View of Dementia." In *Mental Health and Spirituality in Later Life*, edited by Elizabeth MacKinlay, 69–75. New York: Haworth, 2003.

Coleman, Peter G. "Ageing and Personhood in Twenty-first-century Europe: A Challenge to Religion." *International Journal of Public Theology* 3 (2009) 63–77.

Crist, Janice D., and Christine A. Tanner. "Interpretation/Analysis Methods in Hermeneutic Interpretive Phenomenology." *Nursing Research* 52.3 (2003) 202–5.

Davis, Robert. *My Journey into Alzheimer's Disease.* Carol Stream, IL: Tynedale House, 1989.

Dewing, Jan. "Personhood and Dementia: Revisiting Tom Kitwood's Ideas." *International Journal of Older People Nursing* 3 (2008) 3–13.

Doka, Kenneth J. "Disenfranchised Grief in Historical and Cultural Perspective." In *Handbook of Bereavement Research and Practice: Advances in Theory and Interventions*, edited by Margaret Stroebe et al., 223–40. Washington, DC: APA, 2008.

———. "Grief and Dementia." In *Living with Grief: Alzheimer's Disease*, edited by Kenneth J. Doka, 139–54. Washington, DC: Hospice Foundation of America, 2004.

———. "Mourning Psychosocial Loss: Anticipatory Mourning." In *Clinical Dimensions of Anticipatory Mourning: Theory and Practice in Working with the Dying, their Loved Ones, and their Caregivers*, edited by Therese A. Rando, 477–92. Champaign, IL: Research, 2000.

Eisenhandler, Susan A. *Keeping the Faith in Late Life.* New York: Springer, 2003.

Everett, Debbie. "Forget Me Not: The Spiritual Care of People with Alzheimer's Disease." *Journal of Health Care Chaplaincy* 8.1–2 (1998) 77–88.

Exline, Julia Juola, and Ephraim Rose. "Religious and Spiritual Struggles." In *Handbook of the Psychology of Religion and Spirituality*, edited by Raymond F. Paloutzian and Crystal L. Park, 315–30. New York: Guilford, 2005.

Field, Nigel P. "Whether to Relinquish or Maintain Bonds with the Deceased." In *Handbook of Bereavement Research and Practice: Advances in Theory and Interventions*, edited by Margaret Stroebe et al., 113–32. Washington, DC: APA, 2008.

Field, Nigel P., and C. Wogrin. "The Changing Bond in Therapy for Unresolved Loss: An Attachment Theory Perspective." In *Grief and Bereavement in Contemporary Society,* edited by Robert. A. Neimeyer, et al., 37–46. New York: Routledge Taylor & Francis, 2011.

Furnish, Victor Paul. *New Testament Theology: The Theology of the First Letter to the Corinthians*. Cambridge: Cambridge University Press, 1999.

Gillies, James, and Robert Neimeyer. "Loss, Grief and the Search for Significance: Towards a Model of Meaning Reconstruction in Bereavement." *Journal of Constructivist Psychology* 19.1 (2006) 31–65.

Goldsmith, Malcolm. *In a Strange Land: People with Dementia in the Local Church*. Southwell, UK: 4M Publications, 2004.

———. "'They Maintained the Fabric of this World': Spirituality and the Non-religious." In *Spirituality and Personhood in Dementia*, edited by Albert Jewell, 165–74. London: Kingsley, 2011.

Gunton, Colin E. *The Promise of Trinitarian Theology*. Edinburgh: T. & T. Clark, 1991.

Hauerwas, Stanley. *Naming the Silences: God, Medicine and the Problem of Suffering*. Grand Rapids: Eerdmans, 1990.

Holley, Caitlin K., and Benjamin T. Mast. "The Impact of Anticipatory Grief on Caregiver Burden in Dementia Caregivers." *The Gerontologist* 49.3 (2009) 388–96.

Hopson, Ronald E., and Gene Rice. "The Book of *Job* as a Resource for Counseling." *The Journal of Pastoral Care & Counseling* 62.1–2 (2008) 87–98.

Hughes, Julian C., et al. "Ingredients and Issues in Supportive Care for People with Dementia: Summarizing from Models of Care." In *Supportive Care for the Person with Dementia*, edited by Julian C. Hughes et al., 99–104. Oxford: Oxford University Press, 2010.

Jacobson, Rolf. "Burning our Lamps with Borrowed Oil: The Liturgical Use of the Psalms and the Life of Faith." In *Psalms and Practice: Worship, Virtue, and Authority*, edited by Stephen Breck Reid, 90–98. Minnesota, MN: Liturgical, 2001.

Jewell, Albert. "Nourishing the Inner Spirit: A Spirituality Model." In *Ageing, Spirituality and Well-Being*, edited by Albert Jewell, 11–26. London: Kingsley, 2004.

Jewett, Robert, assisted by Roy Kotansky. *Romans: A Commentary*. Edited by Eldon Jay Epp. Minneapolis: Fortress, 2007.

Johnson, Kelly S. "Praying: Poverty." In *The Blackwell Companion to Christian Ethics*, 1st ed., edited by Stanley Hauerwas and Samuel Wells, 225–36. Malden, MA: Blackwell, 2004.

Kenneson, Philip. "Gathering: Worship, Imagination, and Formation." In *The Blackwell Companion to Christian Ethics*, edited by Stanley Hauerwas and Samuel Wells, 53–67. Malden, MA: Blackwell, 2004.

Kidner, Derek. *Psalms 73–150: An Introduction and Commentary on Books III, IV and V of the Psalms*. London: InterVarsity Press, 1975.

Kilby, Karen. "Perichoresis and Projection: Problems with Social Doctrines of the Trinity." *New Blackfriars* 81.956 (2000) 432–55.

Killick, John. "Becoming a Friend of Time: A Consideration of How We May Approach Persons with Dementia through Spiritual Sharing in the Moment." In *Spirituality and Personhood in Dementia*, edited by Albert Jewell, 52–63. London: Kingsley, 2011.

———. "Dementia, Identity and Spirituality." *Journal of Religious Gerontology* 16.3 (2004) 59–74.

———. "Magic Mirrors: What People with Dementia Show Us about Ourselves." In *Ageing, Spirituality and Well-Being*, edited by Albert Jewell, 143–52. London: Kingsley, 2004.

BIBLIOGRAPHY

Killick, John, and Kate Allan. *Communication and the Care of People with Dementia.* Philadelphia: Open University Press, 2001.

Kitwood, Tom. *Dementia Reconsidered: The Person Comes First.* Maidenhead, UK: Open University Press, 1997.

Kontos, Pia C. "Ethnographic Reflections on Selfhood, Embodiment and Alzheimer's Disease." *Ageing and Society* 24.6 (2004) 829–49.

Kotai-Ewers, T. *Listen to the Talk of Us: People with Dementia Speak Out.* Shenton Park, Western Australia: Alzheimer's Australia, 2007.

Krueger, Richard A., and Mary Anne Casey. *Focus Groups: A Practical Guide for Applied Research.* 3rd ed. Thousand Oaks, CA: Sage, 2000.

Larkin, Michael, et al. "Giving Voice and Making Sense in Interpretative Phenomenological Analysis." *Qualitative Research in Psychology* 3 (2006) 102–20.

Latini, Theresa F. "Grief-work in Light of the Cross: Illustrating Transformational Interdisciplinarity." *Journal of Psychology and Theology* 37.2 (2009) 87–95.

Lenshyn, John. "Reaching the Living Echo." *Alzheimer's Care Quarterly* 6.1 (2005) 20–28.

Lyall, David. *Integrity of Pastoral Care.* London: SPCK, 2001.

Lyon, B. "What is the Relevance of Congregational Studies for Pastoral Theology?" In *The Blackwell Reader in Pastoral and Practical Theology*, edited by James Woodward and Stephen Pattison, 257–71. Malden, MA: Blackwell, 2000.

McCarthy, Marie. "Spirituality in a Postmodern Era." In *The Blackwell Reader in Pastoral and Practical Theology*, edited by James Woodward and Stephen Pattison, 192–206. Malden, MA: Blackwell, 2000.

McFadden, Susan H. "Gathering and Growing Gifts through Creative Expression and Playfulness." In *Spirituality and Personhood in Dementia*, edited by Albert Jewell, 100–110. London: Kingsley, 2011.

McFadden, Susan H., and John T. McFadden. *Aging Together: Dementia, Friendship and Flourishing Communities.* Baltimore: Johns Hopkins University Press, 2011.

McGrath, Pam. "Creating a Language for 'Spiritual Pain' through Research: A Beginning." *Support Care Cancer* 10 (2002) 637–46.

MacKinlay, Elizabeth. "Friends and Neighbours: Pastoral Care and Ageing in Christian Perspective." In *Ageing and Spirituality across Faiths and Cultures*, edited by Elizabeth MacKinlay, 68–80. London: Kingsley, 2010.

———. "Walking with a Person into Dementia: Creating Care Together." In *Spirituality and Personhood in Dementia*, edited by Albert Jewell, 42–51. London: Kingsley, 2011.

MacKinlay, Elizabeth, and Corinne Trevitt. *Finding Meaning in the Experience of Dementia: The Place of Spiritual Reminiscence Work.* London: Kingsley, 2012.

Mandolfo, Carleen. *God in the Dock: Dialogic Tension in the Psalms of Lament.* Sheffield, UK: Sheffield Academic Press, 2002.

Marquez-Gonsalez, et al. "Anger, Spiritual Meaning and Support from the Religious Community in Dementia Caregiving." *Journal of Religious Health* 51 (2010) 179–86.

Marris, Peter. "Holding onto Meaning through the Life Cycle." In *Challenges of the Third Age: Meaning and Purpose in Later Life*, edited by Robert S. Weiss and Scott A. Bass, 13–28. Oxford: Oxford University Press, 2002.

Meuser, Thomas M., et al. "Assessing Grief in Family Caregivers." In *Living with Grief: Alzheimer's Disease*, edited by Kenneth Doka, 169–95. Washington, DC: Hospice Foundation of America, 2004.

Bibliography

Mitchell, G., et al. "'Diagnosing' and 'Managing' Spiritual Distress in Palliative Care: Creating an Intellectual Framework for Spirituality Useable in Clinical Practice." *Australasian Medical Journal* 3.6 (2010) 364–69.

Moltmann, Jürgen. *The Crucified God: The Cross of Christ as the Foundation and Criticism of Christian Theology.* Translated by R. A. Wilson and John Bowden. Minneapolis: Fortress, 1993.

Morgan, David. "The Existential Quest for Meaning." In *Death and Spirituality*, edited by Kenneth Doka and David Morgan, 3–10. Amityville, NY: Baywood, 1993.

Morgan, David L. *Focus Groups as Qualitative Research.* 2nd ed. Thousand Oaks, CA: Sage, 1997.

Mowat, Harriet. "Ageing, Health Care and the Spiritual Imperative—A View from Scotland." In, *Successful Ageing, Spirituality and Meaning*, edited by J. Bouwer, 109–20. Leuven: Peeters, 2010.

———."Voicing the Spiritual: Working with People with Dementia." In *Spirituality and Personhood in Dementia*, edited by Albert Jewell, 75–86. London: Kingsley, 2011.

Moyle, Wendy, et al. "Living with Loss: Dementia and the Family Caregiver." *Australian Journal of Advanced Nursing* 19.3 (2002) 25–31.

Neimeyer, Robert A. "The Language of Loss: Grief Therapy as a Process of Meaning Reconstruction." In *Meaning Reconstruction and the Experience of Loss*, edited by Robert A. Neimeyer, 261–92. Washington, DC: APA, 2001.

———, ed. *Meaning Reconstruction and the Experience of Loss.* Washington DC: APA, 2001.

Neimeyer, Robert A., and Adam Anderson. "Meaning Reconstruction Theory." In *Loss and Grief: A Guide to Human Services Practitioners*, edited by Neil Thompson, 45–64. Basingstoke, UK: Palgrave Macmillan, 2002.

Neimeyer, Robert A., and Joseph Currier. "Bereavement Interventions: Present Status and Future Horizons." *Grief Matters* 11.1 (2008) 18–22.

Neimeyer, Robert A., and Louis A. Gamino, "The Experience of Grief and Bereavement." In *Handbook of Death and Dying*, edited by Clifton D. Bryant, 847–54. Thousand Oaks, CA: Sage, 2003.

Neimeyer, Robert A., and J. R Jordan. "Disenfranchisement as Empathic Failure: Grief Therapy and the Co-construction of Meaning." In *Disenfranchised Grief: New Directions, Challenges, and Strategies for Practice*, edited by Kenneth J. Doka, 95–118. Champaign, IL: Research, 2002.

Neimeyer, Robert A., et al. "Mourning and Meaning." *The American Behavioral Scientist* 46.2 (2002) 235–54.

O'Shaughnessy, Margaret, et al. "Changes in the Couple Relationship in Dementia Care." *Dementia* 9.2 (2010) 237–58.

Ozorak, Elizabeth Weiss. "Cognitive Approaches to Religion." In *Handbook of the Psychology of Religion and Spirituality*, 1st ed., edited by Raymond F. Paloutzian and Crystal L. Park, 216–34. New York: Guilford, 2005.

Pargament, Kenneth I. *The Psychology of Religion and Coping: Theory, Research, Practice.* New York: Guilford, 1997.

Pargament, Kenneth I., et al. "The Religious Dimension of Coping." In *Handbook of the Psychology of Religion and Spirituality*, 1st ed., edited by Raymond F. Paloutzian and Crystal L. Park, 479–95. New York: Guilford, 2005.

Bibliography

Park, Crystal L. "Religion and Meaning." In *Handbook of the Psychology of Religion and Spirituality*, 1st ed., edited by Raymond F. Paloutzian and Crystal L. Park, 295-314. New York: Guilford, 2005.

Park, Crystal L., and Roshi Joan Halifax. "Religion and Spirituality in Adjusting to Bereavement: Grief as Burden, Grief as Gift." In *Grief and Bereavement in Contemporary Society: Bridging Research and Practice*, edited by Robert A. Neimeyer et al., 355-63. New York: Routledge Taylor & Francis, 2011.

Park, Crystal L., and Raymond F. Paloutzian. "One Step toward Integration and an Expansive Future." In *Handbook of the Psychology of Religion and Spirituality*, 1st ed., edited by Raymond F. Paloutzian and Crystal L. Park, 550-64. New York: Guilford, 2005.

Pattison, Stephen. *The Challenge of Practical Theology: Selected Essays*. London: Kingsley, 2007.

Pattison, Stephen, with James Woodward. "A Vision of Pastoral Theology: The Search for Words that Resurrect the Dead." In *Spiritual Dimensions of Pastoral Care: Practical Theology in a Multidisciplinary Context*, edited by David Willows and John Swinton, 36-50. London: Kingsley, 2000.

Pembroke, Neil. *Pastoral Care in Worship: Liturgy and Psychology in Dialogue*. London: T. & T. Clark, 2010.

———. *Renewing Pastoral Practice: Trinitarian Perspectives on Pastoral Care and Counselling*. Aldershot, UK: Ashgate, 2006.

———. *Working Relationships: Spirituality in Human Service and Organisational Life*. London: Kingsley, 2004.

Ponder, Rebecca, and Elizabeth Pomeroy. "The Grief of Caregivers: How Pervasive Is It?" *Journal of Gerontological Social Work* 27.1/2 (1996) 3-21.

Post, Stephen G. *The Moral Challenge of Alzheimer's Disease*. Baltimore: Johns Hopkins University Press, 1995.

———. "*Respectare*: Moral Respect for the Lives of the Deeply Forgetful." In *Dementia: Mind, Meaning, and the Person*, edited by Julian Hughes et al., 223-30. Oxford: Oxford University Press, 2006.

Pringle, Jan, et al. "Interpretative Phenomenological Analysis: A Discussion and Critique." *Nurse Researcher* 18.3 (2011) 20-24.

Purves, Andrew. *Reconstructing Pastoral Theology: A Christological Foundation*. Louisville: Westminster John Knox, 2004.

Rando, Therese A. *Treatment of Complicated Mourning*. Champaign, IL: Research, 1993.

Robinson, L., et al. "Making Sense of Dementia and Adjusting to Loss: Psychological Reactions to a Diagnosis of Dementia in Couples." *Aging and Mental Health* 9.4 (2005) 337-47.

Sabat, Steven R. "Maintaining the Self in Dementia." In *Supportive Care for the Person with Dementia*, edited by Julian C. Hughes et al., 227-34. Oxford: Oxford University Press, 2010.

———. "Selfhood and Alzheimer's Disease." In *The Person with Alzheimer's Disease: Pathways to Understanding the Experience*, edited by Phyllis Braudy Harris, 88-111. Baltimore: Johns Hopkins University Press, 2002.

Sanders, Sara, and Kathryn B. Adams. "Grief Reactions and Depression in Caregivers of Individuals with Alzheimer's Disease: Results from a Pilot Study in an Urban Setting." *Health and Social Work* 30.4 (2005) 287-95.

BIBLIOGRAPHY

Sapp, Stephen. "Ethics and Dementia: Dilemmas Encountered by Clergy and Chaplains." In *Aging, Spirituality, and Religion: A Handbook*, Vol. 2., edited by Melvin Kimble and Susan H. McFadden, 355-67. Minneapolis: Fortress, 2002.

———. "Spiritual Care of People with Dementia and Their Carers." In *Supportive Care for the Person with Dementia*, edited by Julian C. Hughes et al., 199-206. Oxford: Oxford University Press, 2010.

Schultz, Cynthia L., and Darcy L. Harris. "Giving Voice to Nonfinite Loss and Grief in Bereavement." In *Grief and Bereavement in Contemporary Society: Bridging Research and Practice*, edited by Robert A. Neimeyer et al., 235-45. New York: Routledge Taylor & Francis, 2011.

Schultz, Noel C. *Forgetting But Not Forgotten*. Adelaide, South Australia: Open Book, 2004.

Settersten, Richard A. "Social Sources of Meaning in Later Life." In *Challenges of the Third Age: Meaning and Purpose in Later Life*, edited by Robert S. Weiss and Scott A. Bass, 55-80. Oxford: Oxford University Press, 2002.

Shamy, Eileen. *A Guide to the Spiritual Dimension of Care for People with Alzheimer's Disease and Related Dementia: More than Body, Brain and Breath*. London: Kingsley, 2003.

Shear, M. Katherine, et al., "Treating Complicated Grief: Converging Approaches." In *Grief and Bereavement in Contemporary Society: Bridging Research and Practice*, edited by Raymond A. Neimeyer, et al., 139-62. New York: Routledge Taylor and Francis, 2011.

Sheard, David. "Bringing Relationships into the Heart of Dementia Care." *Journal of Dementia Care* July/August (2004) 22-24.

Shenk, David. *The Forgetting: Alzheimer's: Portrait of an Epidemic*. Toronto: Random House, 2002.

Simpkins, Daphne. *The Long Goodnight: My Father's Journey into Alzheimer's*. Grand Rapids: Eerdmans, 2003.

Small, Neil, et al. "Improving End-of-Life Care for People with Dementia." In *Caregiving in Dementia: Research and Applications* Vol. 4, edited by Bere M. L. Miesen and Gemma M. M. Jones, 365-92. London: Brunner-Routledge, 2006.

Smith, Jonathan A., et al. *Interpretative Phenomenological Analysis: Theory, Method and Research*. Los Angeles: Sage, 2009.

Snyder, Lisa. "Satisfactions and Challenges in Spiritual Faith and Practice for Persons with Dementia." *Dementia* 2 (2003) 299-308.

———. *Speaking our Minds*. New York: Freeman, 1999.

Speck, Peter. "Dementia and Spiritual Care." In *Caregiving in Dementia: Research and Applications* Vol. 4, edited by Bere M. L. Miesen and Gemma M. M. Jones, 241-56. London: Brunner-Routledge, 2006.

Stokes, Graham. "From Psychological Interventions to a Psychology of Dementia." In *Supportive Care for the Person with Dementia*, edited by Julian C. Hughes et al., 159-70. Oxford: Oxford University Press, 2010.

Stroebe, Margaret S., and Henk Schut. "The Dual Process Model of Coping with Bereavement: Overview and Update." *Grief Matters* 11.1 (2008) 4-10.

Swinton, John. "Being in the Moment: Developing a Contemplative Approach to Spiritual Care with People who have Dementia." In *Spirituality and Personhood in Dementia*, edited by Albert Jewell, 175-85. London: Kingsley, 2011.

———. *Dementia: Living in the Memories of God*. Grand Rapids: Eerdmans, 2012.

Bibliography

———. "Forgetting Whose We Are—Theological Reflections on Successful Ageing, Personhood and Dementia." In *Successful Ageing, Spirituality and Meaning: Multidisciplinary Perspectives*, edited by J. Bouwer, 237–62. Leuven: Peeters, 2010.

———. *Spirituality and Mental Health Care: Rediscovering a "Forgotten" Dimension*. London: Kingsley, 2001.

Swinton, John, and Harriet Mowat. *Practical Theology and Qualitative Research*. London: SCM, 2006.

Thornton, Sharon B. *Broken yet Beloved: A Pastoral Theology of the Cross*. St. Louis, MO: Chalice, 2002.

Trevitt, Corinne, and Elizabeth MacKinlay. "'I am Just an Ordinary Person . . .': Spiritual Reminiscence in Older People with Memory Loss." In *Aging, Spirituality and Palliative Care*, edited by Elizabeth MacKinlay, 79–91. New York: Haworth, 2006.

Vanier, Jean. *The Broken Body: Journey to Wholeness*. London: Darton, Longman and Todd, 1988.

Veling, Terence. *Practical Theology: On Earth as It is in Heaven*. Maryknoll, NY: Orbis, 2005.

Villanueva, Federico G. *The 'Uncertainty of a Hearing': A Study of the Sudden Change of Mood in the Psalms of Lament*. Leiden: Brill, 2008.

Walter, Tony. "A New Model of Grief: Bereavement and Biography." *Mortality: Promoting the InterDisciplinary Study of Death and Dying* 1.1 (1996) 7–25.

Wilkinson, Sue. "Focus Group Research." In *Qualitative Research: Theory, Method and Practice*, 2nd ed., edited by David Silverman, 177–99. London: Sage, 2004.

Witherington, Ben. *Conflict and Community in Corinth: A Socio-rhetorical Commentary on 1 and 2 Corinthians*. Grand Rapids: Eerdmans, 1995.

Worden, J. William. *Grief Counseling and Grief Therapy: A Handbook for the Mental Health Practitioner*. New York: Springer, 2002.

Zinnbauer, Brian J., and Kenneth I. Pargament. "Religiousness and Spirituality." In *Handbook of the Psychology of Religion and Spirituality*, edited by Raymond F. Paloutzian and Crystal L. Park, 21–42. New York: Guilford, 2005.

Zylla, Phil C. *The Roots of Sorrow: A Pastoral Theology of Suffering*. Waco, TX: Baylor University Press, 2012.

Index

A
advocacy (advocate), x, xxi, 95, 127, 155, 184–86, 191, 193–94
Allan, Kate, 11, 105
Allen, Brian, 27
Allford, Judith, 28
Anderson, Ray, 16, 21
ambiguity (ambiguous),
    in caregivers' experience, 37, 41, 51–52, 57, 59, 74, 79–80, 91–93, 96–97
    and Christian experience, 161–62
    in dementia-related loss, *see* loss(es), ambiguous
    support in, 105–8, 187, 192, 194
ambivalence,
    in caregivers' experience, 37, 41, 51–52, 54–55, 59, 87
    and loss, 105, 110, 114
analysis, interpretive,
    of caregiver research data, 36–39, 40–43, 46–48, 51–54, 57–61, 63–66, 90–99
    of local practice research data, 137–54
analysis, thematic,
    of caregiver research data, 68–90
    of local practice research data, 122–35
anger,
    in caregivers' experience, 28, 36–37, 51, 53–54, 56, 59, 63, 72–73, 79, 92, 94, 192
    in families, 110
    towards God, 20, 160–61, 164
    and persons with dementia, 8, 133
anguish, 106, 160–61, 163–64
attitudes, dehumanizing, 2–3

B
Baldwin, Clive, 8, 9, 12
Barth, Karl, 7, 16
Bender, Michael, 10, 109–10
Boden, Christine, 25
body,
    "body of Christ," xix, xxi, 117, 156–58, 163, 167–68, 170, 172–73, 177–81, 183, 191–92, 195
    and dementia, 5–7, 11, 15, 29, 41, 74, 130
    local practice research and "body of Christ," 127, 136, 144, 152
    theology of, 7, 15, 29, 191–92
Boss, Pauline, 41, 105–6, 110
Bramble, Marguerite, et al., 14
Brennan, Tim, 28
Brueggemann, Walter, 162
Bryden, Christine, 25, 111, 182, 184
Bryden, Christine, and Elizabeth MacKinlay, 25, 27, 117
Bryden, Christine with Sarah Minns, 25

Index

C

care,
    communicative, 2, 11–12, 28, 191
    empathic, (*see* empathy)
    narrative supportive, 12–14
    person-centered, xix, 2, 3, 8–10, 15, 28, 190
    relational, ix, xix, 2, 8–10, 15–16, 28, 182, 191
    supportive, 8, 10, 12–13, 16, 28, 190
care, pastoral,
    caregivers' experience of, 40, 43, 53, 62, 65, 67, 85–86, 116, 176–77
    in Christian community, 156–57, 163, 166–68, 172–74, 177–79, 182–86, 195
    and dementia, xviii–xix, xxi, 1–2, 14–16, 28, 34, 174–75, 181–84, 189, 195
    and hope, 14, 113–116, 156–57, 175–76, 183–85
    and reciprocity, 179, 189
    and suffering, 116
care, spiritual,
    and dementia, xvii, xix–xx, 22–29, 96–97, 99, 113–15, 155, 184–85, 194
    and grief work, 113–15
    in holistic care, 9, 15, 17, 20–22
    and listening, *see* listening 192–93, 195
Coleman, Peter, 21, 64
comfort,
    in Christian community, 136–37, 163, 167–69, 179, 184, 193
    false, 163
    God's, 166–69, 195
    for persons with dementia, 8, 13, 22
    spiritual, 20–21, 114
communication,
    in caregivers' experience, 40, 91, 97
    and care, *see* care, communicative
    and Christian community, 179–80
    with persons with dementia, xiv, 6–7, 11–12, 21–23, 114, 179, 183
community,
    Christian, xviii–xix, xxi, 6, 16, 19, 27–28, 98, 101, 154–164, 167–82, 185–86, 190–92, 195
    spiritual, 18–19, 27–28, 154
companion,
    empathic, 1–2, 13, 104, 192–93
    listening, 24–25
    pastoral, 182–84, 189
    spiritual, xxi, 103, 182–84
companionship, loss of, in caregivers' experience, 41, 50–51, 58, 68, 75, 93, 108, 161–62
compassion,
    in Christian community, xix–xix, 101, 159, 164–69, 171–73, 179–81, 187, 195
    of God, 144, 159, 165–69, 176, 193, 195
    and meaning-making, 114
    and spiritual caregiving, 20, 23, 194
    withholding of, 167
conflict,
    in beliefs, 20, 113, 161, 164, 173
    in emotions, 105
    in family, 14, 105
    and spiritual care, 22, 28
coping,
    in caregiver research, 37, 41–42, 47–48, 52, 55, 59–60, 68, 72, 80–83, 87–88, 97, 99
    and grief, 41, 106, 109, 111, 113–14, 192
    and help-seeking, 178
    and meaning-making, 19–20, 28–29
    and spiritual care, 22, 28, 184
"coping mode," 127, 142
counter-story, 1–2, 13, 183–84, 194
Crist, Janice and Christine Tanner, 32, 34

Index

D
Davis, Robert, 164
Dewing, Jan, 3
dementia
    and communication, *see* communication
    and creativity, 6, 21–23, 26–27, 193
    and emotions, 10–12, 27, 110–14
    and identity, *see* identity
    and malignant social positioning, 2–3, 8–10, 100, 178
    and narrative, *see* narrative
    and relationships, *see* relationship(s)
    and spirituality, *see* spirituality
    and worship, *see* worship
disappointment,
    in caregivers' experience, 41, 59, 72, 155
    about support, 19, 28, 57, 83
dissonance, cognitive, 164
distress(ed),
    in caregivers' experience, 35–38, 41, 50, 60, 72–73, 75, 79, 92
    and faith, 20, 163
    in grief, 108–9, 123–24, 126, 140, 147, 183–84
    of person(s) with dementia, 124, 131
    spiritual, 20–21, 29, 39, 60, 113–14, 185, 193
Doka, Kenneth, 58, 105, 107–8

E
Eisenhandler, Susan, 19, 32, 97
emotions,
    caregivers' experience of, 30, 33, 36–38, 42, 48, 61–63, 66, 72, 79–80, 82, 91–92, 94–96, 99, 155
    Christian approach(es) to, 160–61, 163–64, 179–80, 182–83, 188
    in grief, 104–5, 109–10
empathy (empathic),
    care, 2, 12, 158
    caregivers' experience of, 38, 43, 58, 60, 67, 85–86, 95–96, 155, 167
    in Christian communities, 158, 160, 165, 174–75, 178–79, 187, 192–93, 195
    failure *see* failure, empathic
    and grief, 95, 104, 115, 187
    listening, 95, 114, 174–75, 180, 189, 194
    local practice research and, 136, 139, 155, 167
    of persons with dementia, 13
    relationship, 24, 114–15, 178–79, 183, 189, 193, 195
Everett, Debbie, 27
Exline, Julia Juola, and Ephraim Rose, 20

F
failure, empathic, 96, 105, 107, 112, 155, 180, 194
Field, Nigel, 102
Field, Nigel, and C. Wogrin, 102
focus group methodology, *see* methodology
friendship(s),
    caregivers' experience of, 43, 57–58, 64, 93, 98, 155
    in Christian community, xxi, 158–59, 173, 179–80, 184–89, 191
    Jesus' model of, 159, 185
    in local practice research, 123–24, 126, 131, 136, 139, 141
    pastoral, 147, 159
Furnish, Victor, 157

G
Gillies, James, and Robert Neimeyer, 103
Goldsmith, Malcolm, 14, 22, 25
"Goodbye, My Mother," 197–99
Gunton, Colin E., 4

grief,
    and ambiguous loss, *see* ambiguity
    anticipatory, 108–9, 113, 115
    in caregivers' experience, 37, 51–52, 77–79, 91–94; for persons with dementia, 100, 111
    and chronic sorrow, 92, 106–7, 112, 194
    complicated, 94, 102–5, 108
    disenfranchised, 105, 107–8, 113–15, 194, in caregivers' experience, 57–59, 68, 155
    and identity, *see* identity
    and meaning-making, 66, 103–7, 109–15
    of persons with dementia, 100–101, 110–11
grief theory (bereavement), 100–104
    application in dementia, 104, 111–12
    continuing bonds, 102
    dual process model, 102
    meaning-making, 103–4
    single pathway models, 101–2

H
Hauerwas, Stanley, 161, 167
Holley, Caitlin K., and Benjamin T. Mast, 109
hope(s),
    in caregivers' experience, 57–58, 60, 62, 66, 83, 105, 160, 184
    and Christian community, xxi, 136, 144, 155–60, 168–71, 173–76, 188, 195
    in grief, 102, 105–6, 114–16
    meta-narrative of, 13–14, 115–16
    and pastoral care, *see* care, pastoral
    of persons with dementia, 12, 22–24, 26
hopelessness (loss of hope), 58, 60, 66, 88, 96, 107, 133
Hopson, Ronald E., and Gene Rice, 162
hospitality, xxi, 154, 158–59, 179–80, 187, 191, 193
Hughes, Julian C., 10

I
identity,
    in caregivers' experience, 38, 41, 47, 52–53, 57–60, 63–64, 74, 77, 93–95, 154
    in Christ, 175, 179–80, 182
    in Christian community, 154, 169–71, 174–75, 180, 189, 192–93
    couple-, 109, 187
    and dementia, xix–xx, 1, 5, 8–10, 12–13, 15, 24–26, 29, 109–10, 175, 182–83, 187, 192–94
    and grief, 100, 103–4, 106, 112
    loss of, 5, 13, 28, 109, 112, 154
    and meaning-making, 94–95, 112–13
    and narrative, 12, 13, 114, 180, 192
    personal, 9–10, 15, 103, 183
    and religion/spirituality, 18–19, 24–26, 113, 115
    social, 93, 110, 187
    theology of, 5–6, 175
imagination,
    empathic, 11–12, 179, 189
    ironic, 175
    social, 171
    of persons with dementia, 27
indifference, in Christian community, 155, 165, 167–68, 179, 192, 195
interdependence,
    in Christian community, xxi, 157–58, 170, 172, 177–79, 181, 188–89, 191, 193, 195
    in "I-Thou" relationship, 8
isolation,
    caregivers' experience of, 28, 38, 43, 51, 55, 60–61, 64, 66–67, 75, 86, 92–93, 192, 194
    and caregiver grief, 109, 113

Index

and Christian community, 176, 180, 188
of persons with dementia, 23, 151, 158, 164, 184, 190
reduction of, 10, 108–9, 176, 180, 184, 188, 194
in suffering, 161–62, 164

J
Jacobson, Rolf, 164
Jewell, Albert, 17–18, 21

K
Kitwood, Tom, 3, 8, 9
Kontos, Pia C., 6
Kotai-Ewers, T., 24

L
lament, xxi, 160–61, 163–64, 181–83
Larkin, Michael et al., 31–32
Latini, Theresa F., 166
Lenshyn, John, 26
listening,
    caregivers' views on, 43, 59, 85, 87, 90, 96, 98
    in Christian community, 175, 179–80, 192, 194–95
    empathic, 104, 114, 180, 183, 194
    and identity, 183, 194
    in local practice research, 127, 133, 136, 139–40, 149–50
    and loss, 23, 104, 109–11, 127, 183, 192
    and meaning-making, 110, 174–75
    and narrative, 14, 180
    to persons with dementia, 11, 13–14, 23, 26, 110–11, 127, 192, 194
    in spiritual care, 114, 183, 194
loneliness, 14, 20, 38, 153, 164, 188
    in caregivers' experience, 58–60, 62–64, 67, 81, 91–93, 95–96, 160, 192
    in Christian community, 160–61, 167
    and persons with dementia, 124
    in suffering, 19, 154, 160–61, 167
loss(es),
    ambiguous, xiii, 105–9, 111–15, 187, 194
    in caregivers' experience, 14, 28, 37–41, 50–52, 55–61, 65–68, 73–80, 82, 90–97, 99–100, 154–55, 192
    in Christian community, 176, 178, 180, 183–84, 187–88, 193
    and dementia, xvii, xxi, 6, 8–9, 13–16, 23–24, 28, 108–15, 158, 164, 192, 197
    and narrative, see narrative of loss
    nonfinite, 107, 112–15
    and persons with dementia, 5, 11, 23–26, 100, 110–11, 175, 182–84
    and support, 14, 104–6, 108–10, 113–16, 187, 194
love,
    agape xxi, 157–59, 166, 177–78, 188, 191–92
    relational, of God, xxi, 16, 190, 195
Lyall, David, 156, 159, 166, 168
Lyon, B., 156

M
McCarthy, Marie, 18, 174
McFadden, Susan H., 27, 182
McFadden, Susan H., and John T. McFadden, 21, 23, 154, 158
MacKinlay, Elizabeth, 23–24, 159, 182
MacKinlay, Elizabeth and Corinne Trevitt, 12–13, 17, 19, 24, 111
McGrath, Pam, 20
Mandolfo, Carleen, 161
Marquez-Gonsalez et al., 53
Marris, Peter, 19, 57
meaning(s),
    in caregivers' experience, 31–34, 38–39, 42, 45–46, 49–50, 58, 60, 64, 66, 68, 88–92, 94–97

Index

meaning(s) (*continued*),
    global and situational, 19–20, 94, 96, 189
    search for, 17–20, 28, 60, 103, 107
    and spirituality, *see* spirituality
meaning-making,
    and aging, 21
    in community, 174–75, 187, 193–94
    and grief, *see* grief
    and persons with dementia, 6, 13–14, 24–25, 27–29
    and spirituality, xix, 19–22, 28, 38, 96, 106, 112–15
method(ology),
    of focus group research, 118–22
    of interpretive phenomenological analysis, 30–34
Meuser, Thomas M., et al., 109
Mitchell, G., et al., 20
model,
    of community care, 22
    of grief, *see* grief
    Jesus' (model) of friendship, 159
    Jesus' (model) of ministry, 144
    medical, 3, 13, 28
    of pastoral care, x, 154–57, 189, 193–95
    of spirituality, 18
Moltmann, Jurgen, 166
Morgan, David, 18, 22
Morgan, David L., 118
Mowat, Harriet, 22–24
Moyle, Wendy, et al., 14

N

narrative,
    in caregiver research, 28, 41, 46, 72, 79, 91, 94–96, 114
    Christian, 115–16, 157, 167, 170–73, 175–76
    and dementia, 8, 10, 12–14, 19, 111, 113–14, 170, 180
    and loss, 102–4, 106–7, 110–15
    in pastoral counseling, 13
    personal, 19, 103–4, 114
    religious, 19, 105
    spiritual, 113–15
neglect(ed),
    and Christian community, 154, 158, 178, 181, 192
    in local practice research, 131, 143, 152
    of persons with dementia, 3
Neimeyer, Robert, 103
Neimeyer, Robert, et al., 104
    and Adam Anderson, 94, 103
    and Joseph Currier, 94, 106
    and Louis A. Gamino, 104
    and J. R. Jordan, 92, 104, 107

O

Ozorak, Elizabeth Weiss, 19

P

Pargament, Kenneth I., 19, 65, 97
Pargament, Kenneth I., et al., 19–20
Park, Crystal L., 19–20
Park, Crystal L., and Roshi Joan Halifax, 113
Pattison, Stephen G., 160; with James Woodward, xviii
Pembroke, Neil, 12–13, 158–59, 166, 169, 171–72, 175, 181, 183
person(s),
    embodied, xix, 1, 4, 6–7, 9–10, 15–17, 191
    relational, xix, 1, 4, 15, 17, 190, 192, 194
personhood,
    bestowal of, xix, 2–4, 178, 190–91
    of persons with dementia, 1–3
    and spirituality, 22
    sustenance of, xx, 2, 5, 7–10, 27–29, 114–15, 176, 193–94
    theology of, xix, 2, 4–7, 15–16, 29, 191
phenomenology, interpretive, *see* methodology
Ponder, Rebecca, and Elizabeth Pomeroy, 108
positioning,
    malignant social, 9

negative self-, 9
Post, Stephen, 2
prayer,
  in caregivers' experience, 39–42, 50, 53, 55, 59, 62, 64–65, 80, 83, 85, 87, 97–98, 155
  in Christian community, xxi, 62, 87, 172–74, 179, 181–83, 189, 193
  and identity, 97
  in local practice research, 123–25, 128, 133–37, 139, 141, 148
  and person(s) with dementia, xiii–xiv, 26, 117, 182
Pringle, Jan, et al., 30–32
profiles, caregivers', 33–36, 39–40, 44–45, 49–50, 54–57, 61–62
program, interchurch, x, xxi, 186–88, 193–94
purpose(s),
  and aging, 19
  in caregivers' experience, 39, 41–42, 46, 52, 54, 62, 65–66, 68, 84, 89, 94–97, 104, 155
  God's, xvii–xviii, 171
  and grief, 104, 113–14
  and spiritual care, 17, 21–22, 113–14
Purves, Andrew, 156, 166, 168, 179

R
Rando, Theresa A., 101–2
relationship(s)
  in Christian community, 117, 158–59, 169–70, 174–75, 177–79, 183–85, 187, 189
  and dementia, xix–xx, 2–3, 6–15, 22–26, 29, 108–9, 111–12, 114–15
  in the Godhead, 4, 166
  God-human, 4–6, 15–16, 29, 156, 159
reminiscence,
  and grief, 104, 110–11
  spiritual, 13–14, 24, 183, 187
rituals,
  in grief, 104, 107, 113–14, 188
  in worship, 26, 60, 171–72, 181, 183
Robinson, L., et al., 109, 111

S
Sabat, Steven R., 8–9, 169
Sanders, Sara, and Kathryn B. Adams, 52
Sapp, Stephen, 3, 17
Schultz, Cynthia, and Darcy L. Harris, 107
Schultz, Noel C., 26, 28
self(hood),
  in Christian community, 27, 117, 169–71, 174
  and dementia, 2, 5–10, 12–15, 23–28, 65–66, 92, 94–95, 100, 109–12, 117
  embodied, 6–7
  and grief, 94–95, 101–104, 110–12
  "loss of," in caregivers' experience, 36, 41, 57, 59–60, 65–66, 77
  multi-dimensional, 9–10, 15
self-giving, 159, 171, 178–79, 188
self-identity, 18, 94–95, 104, 109
self-narrative, 103–4
self-stereotyping, negative, 8–9
Settersten, Richard A., 98
Shamy, Eileen, 25–26, 28, 181
Shear, M., Katherine, et al., 103
Sheard, David, 10
Shenk, David, 5
Simpkins, Daphne, 5
Smith, Jonathan A., et al., 31
Snyder, Lisa, 5, 23–24
sorrow, 100, 154, 192
  chronic, 92, 106–7, 112, 194
Speck, Peter, 20
spirituality,
  and dementia, 22–28, 115, 182, 191
  and grief, 113, 115
  and meaning-making, *see* meaning-making
  model of, 17–18
  and religion, 18–19

Index

spirituality (*continued*),
    and support, 21–22, 184, 194
stereotyping, 2, 8, 11, 132, 190
Stokes, Graham, 3
stranger(s), 158–60, 165, 185, 188, 191
stress,
    in caregivers' experience, 14, 35–36, 39, 45, 48, 56, 63, 70, 76, 96, 99, 185
    and grief, 102, 105–6, 109–10
    and meaning-making, 19–20, 95–96
    and support, 19, 187, 194
suffering,
    of Christ, 165–66, 168–69, 175
    in Christian community, xxi, 146, 151, 154–58, 161–65, 167–69, 174–76, 178–82, 185, 188–89, 193
    and grief, 19–21, 113, 115
    and lament, *see* lament
    and loneliness, *see* loneliness
    and pastoral care, 115–16, 166, 182–83
    theology of, 164–69, 173–74
Swinton, John, 1, 3–7, 9–10, 22, 24–27, 157–58, 160, 170, 175
Swinton, John, and Harriet Mowat, 17, 31

T

theology, 3, 128, 147,
    and dementia, xv, 1, 3–7, 22, 26, 170, 175
    of personhood, *see* personhood, theology of
    practical, xv, xvii–xviii, 1, 190, 195
    of suffering, *see* suffering
    Trinitarian, 4

Thornton, Sharon B., xviii
Trinity (Triune God), 4, 16, 157–59, 167, 189, 191

V

Vanier, Jean, 177
Veling, Terence, xvii
Villanueva, Federico, 161

W

Walter, Tony, 103–4
Wilkinson, Sue, 118–19
Witherington, Ben, 157
Worden, J. William, 101, 104
world(s), assumptive,
    in caregivers' experience, 58–60, 63, 65, 91, 94–95
    challenge to, 19–21, 28–29, 114
    Christian, 164, 181
    and grief, 94, 103, 107, 114
worship,
    caregivers' experience of, 39, 42, 53, 62, 83, 86, 98, 155
    inclusive, 180–82, 185, 188
    and lament, 163–64
    local practice and, 123, 127, 130, 134, 136, 142–43, 147–48
    and persons with dementia, 26, 181, 185, 188, 192–93
    and rituals, *see* rituals

Z

Zinnbauer, Brian J., and Kenneth I. Pargament, 18
Zylla, Phil, 154, 160–61, 163, 165, 167, 174

www.ingramcontent.com/pod-product-compliance
Lightning Source LLC
Chambersburg PA
CBHW032057230426
43662CB00035B/586